MATT

AND THE

PORN FREE RADIO PODCAST

FANTASTIC PERSPECTIVE ON BECOMING PORN FREE
★★★★★

Instead of talking about the chemistry and neuroscience of what porn may or may not do to your brain, Matt emphasizes our innate desire for connection and that our porn habits aren't simply physical but they fill some internal, emotional need. Matt is confronting in the sense that he asks what the pain in your life is that porn helps you soothe. How does it comfort you? I resisted this idea, but I've come to realize that I do need to confront these questions. —SJ

POWERFUL
★★★★★

I'm extremely grateful for Matt and his dedication to the message of recovery in compulsive porn use. It takes a lot of passion and vulnerability to discuss these topics and to bring to the table the authenticity that Matt does.

I've learned more about love for myself and shame resilience. I have also learned a plethora of recovery tools that I feel give me so much strength and knowledge in dealing with my own addictions. Totally worth your time. —gollygeewizards

HERE'S THE HELP YOU NEED!
★★★★★

If you have tried unsuccessfully to quit porn, this is the podcast for you! Through his completely nonjudgmental, down-to-earth approach, Matt lays down guidance and helpful tips that really work in the quest to live a life that is free of compulsive porn use! —Sober_Guy05

HOPE FOR EVERYONE
★★★★★

This podcast is the most redemptive, vulnerable, practical, challenging, and hopeful resource I have ever encountered on pornography addiction.

Matt is the boldest, most consistent, most compassionate guide in the journey toward recovery. There are not enough words of gratitude that I have for him and his honesty and hard work in this podcast and the resources he makes available.

If you are believing the lie that there is no hope for you in your addiction, as I had for so long, this podcast is for you. There is hope. There is recovery. And there is new life. For everyone. —Hoosiersman

AUTHENTIC, MOTIVATING, AND INTELLIGENT
★★★★★

Matt is so sincere and real in every episode. Love his stories and this podcast is a real reason why I'm able to stay sober lately. I listen daily. —Jeff H.

HOPEFUL AND ACTION ORIENTED
★★★★★

Thank you for this podcast. It has truly changed my perspective on recovery and is already starting to pay dividends in my life. —Luke2116

MATT SPEAKS THE TRUTH
★★★★★

Awesome programming; I never thought there would be so many relevant topics in the context of porn use and its pitfalls, but Matt brings them all under the umbrella in a logical and entertaining way. There's a religious undertone, but it's employed judiciously and only adds to the show's effectiveness. —Paul G.

WOW!!
★★★★★

It literally feels like Matt is speaking directly to my core. —whiskeysgt1

GREAT INFORMATION
★★★★★

This podcast has really good information for anyone. Whether you are one day sober or one hundred, Matt tackles topics that are relevant and interesting. It has been a wonderful addition to my recovery journey, and I highly recommend it to anyone else on their journey. —Richard186177

THE BEST
★★★★★

The most practical and helpful podcast for recovery from porn. Provides genuine action steps and options to create a road map to sobriety. —Complex7

SUPER GREAT PODCAST
★★★★★

I started listening shortly after disclosing my porn addiction to my wife of eighteen years and Matt has been a big part in my sobriety of one year and two months. I have probably listened to over one hundred episodes. I can sense that Matt has his heart in the right place, and I love his openness, his vulnerability, and the wisdom he is sharing. His podcasts are hands on with many helpful practical tips as well as deeper mental and spiritual guidance and advice. —Rasa1974

GOLD GOLD GOLD!!!
★★★★★

Best podcast I've heard for recovery in the area of purity. —Dave from Orlando

FRESH AIR
★★★★★

Great, realistic information that encourages listeners and provides a road map to freedom. —TBaynes6G

GREAT ADVICE
★★★★★

His ideas and tools surpass most of what I got from therapists. Recommend it to anyone needing help. —Vizual1

GREAT CONTENT WITH USEFUL ACTION STEPS
★★★★★

I have listened to *many* podcasts on this subject, read about twenty books and two hundred articles, attended twelve-step groups regularly, an have been meeting with a counselor for a long time, so I feel that I know what I'm talking about when I say that this guy is more helpful than anything else I've tried. This guy gives great explanations of what is happening and why, and then he gives concrete action items for you to perform to help you overcome this addiction. —jwickwick

THANKFUL FOR THIS PODCAST!
★★★★★

Matt does an amazing job of providing insight and wisdom into the porn recovery journey. I've learned so much about myself and how to identify and overcome triggers and edging behaviors. I highly recommend this podcast for anyone looking for freedom and recovery from porn. —Dwilly23

LIFE CHANGING
★★★★★

Can a podcast be life changing? In this case, YES! I'm so thankful for Matt and his practical applications to fight this horrible addiction. So glad I found this a year ago! —Sec11164

LOVE THE PODCAST!
★★★★★

This is a great podcast for those who are searching for practical wisdom in how to avoid pornography and other forms of acting out sexually. I highly recommend this for anyone that is struggling and looking for help and encouragement. —cdogbrink

LOVE IT
★★★★★

The tools and tips that Matt provides every week have really helped me in my recovery efforts, especially around "being seen" letting others into my life and sharing openly. He has helped me break out of shame and isolation. —philoscr

GREAT SPEAKER WITH MUCH NEEDED MESSAGE
★★★★★

WOW . . . this man is such an inspiration and role model for those who aspire to live a porn-free life. I have struggled with porn for years and have never been able to overcome it. Through the motivating words of wisdom from Matt, I am taking the necessary steps in order to beat this addiction. —Ravens4thewin

BRUTALLY HONEST!
★★★★★

I found this podcast by accident and was immediately taken aback by the honesty of this great man. You can feel the sincerity and truth come through in each episode. —Farmboybeau2

THIS CAN CHANGE YOUR LIFE!
★★★★★

If this is something you have struggled with and need help— DOWNLOAD THIS NOW. Do not put it off, do not wait for your life to change. Whether you are deep in a struggle and don't know where to start or need ongoing encouragement to know what you are fighting for, this is an absolutely amazing series. Matt had the courage to share his story with the rest us and has made us realize we are not alone in this struggle. The podcasts are informative, practical and powerful. This has helped me tremendously— and believe me when I say, if it can help me, it can certainly help you! —ECMidwesterner

AMAZING VULNERABILITY
★★★★★

Matt has done an incredible job of telling it like it is so that we can get past the shame and really work on the root causes. —CAppreciative Man

REFRESHING IDEAS
★★★★★

Matt put things in a new light. One that has really helped reenergize my recovery. —Looking4help

HE KNOWS THE SCHEMES

★★★★★

I've never heard anyone speak so openly about porn addiction. He mentions all the schemes we have thought of and employed and the edges we like to walk up to before we fall. Refreshingly honest and upfront. —Queesho

AMAZINGLY HELPFUL

★★★★★

Originally I thought about how a podcast could do anything for me and my struggle, but after taking a try at listening to it, I have been so surprised in finding this so helpful. Matt is an amazing speaker and never fails to hit the mark on what I need to hear. Matt has helped me to see deeper into the real problems that were keeping me in my addiction and also provides practical ways to fight it. I'm finally able to see a light at the end of the tunnel. I totally recommend this to anyone struggling with pornography. —Carrotman99

POWERFUL TOOL

★★★★★

This podcast is a powerful tool to get you on the road to sobriety. It has helped me tremendously. —Orbalisk

A WINNER!

★★★★★

Matt's authenticity, vulnerability, and talent for storytelling makes this one of the best new podcasts I've heard this year. —Charles777777

MY FAVORITE RECOVERY PODCAST!!!

★★★★★

I love this podcast and have learned lots of recovery tools so far! Today I am doing the best I have ever been in my life in making positive improvements in myself and relationships and in my recovery. I have been addicted for twelve years and I finally see the light at the end of the tunnel and that full recovery is possible! —Cameron (grateful recovering husband)

PORN FREE

BECOMING THE TYPE OF MAN WHO DOES NOT LOOK AT PORN

MATT DOBSCHUETZ

HOST OF THE PORN FREE RADIO PODCAST

TWO FALLS
PUBLISHING

Paperback ISBN: 9781737893202
Hardback ISBN: 9781737893233
eBook ISBN: 9781737893219

SEL041040 SELF-HELP / Compulsive Behavior / Sex & Pornography Addiction
SEL041000 SELF-HELP / Compulsive Behavior / General
SOC034000 SOCIAL SCIENCE / Pornography

Front cover design by Jason Clement
Photos by Jennifer Schuman
Edited by Melissa Miller
Typeset by Kaitlin Barwick

CONTENTS

CONTENTS

INTRODUCTION

I TYPICALLY DON'T HAVE CALLS FIRST thing on Monday morning in my coaching practice, because guys are usually unavailable to talk then. So I was surprised when David scheduled an intro call right after I dropped my kids off at the bus stop.

He quickly told me that in the past week, two things had captured his attention. He had read in the local paper about a prominent businessman getting busted for underage porn. Then on Sunday, as he sat in a pew with his wife, the church announced that one of the leaders had stepped down from his ministry due to pornography.

It was a wake-up call for David, who was struggling with looking at porn at work. His office was walking distance from his house, so he rarely drove to work if it was nice out. He told me that every day on the way to work, he would pray to God, asking to help him not look at pornography that day at work.

But as the stress and tedium of work kicked in, David would find it tougher and tougher to resist. It sometimes was a quick peek at some pictures on Twitter. Other times, on a long boring conference call, he might watch a video. He took some steps to prevent using porn. He asked his IT guy to install a blocker on his PC. That worked for a while, but eventually David found his way around the software.

And it didn't stay at work. When he got home, there were more challenges. The smart TV in the basement that he watched on the treadmill. His wife's laptop. At home, he found it was easy to disappear and go deeper.

He had never really talked about it with anyone except for his wife. Even though his wife cared deeply for him, it was hard to be honest with her. He didn't want to hurt her.

Slips with porn can be very confusing and painful. I think a lot of partners have a nagging question in the back of their mind: "If he loves me and knows this hurts me, why would he go back to it?" After the emotional fallout from a confession or two, David just resolved to hide. To double-down on his self-reliance to stop.

What I remember from the call was how alone David seemed. He was motivated to stop looking at porn but had no idea how. His attempts to stop on his own were one failure after another. This pattern of failure was undermining his confidence. He was feeling hopeless.

On the outside David was a success. He owned a successful business. He ran marathons. He volunteered his time at church. He was a loving father and husband.

But on the inside, he was hurting. He was unable to manage his feelings and compulsion with porn. He felt cut off from others with no road map to recovery. He never looked deeper into what was driving the behavior though. He just *tried* to stop. He made resolutions. He prayed. And he kept going back to porn.

Now, I have had several hundred intake calls like this. But I remember this one clearly. *David was motivated.*

You might not relate to all the details in David's situation, but as we often say in my recovery groups: "The lyrics are different, but the melody is the same." The details of our struggle may vary, but the feelings and the patterns are similar.

When our attempts to stop looking at porn fail, our confidence is shot. We isolate and start living two lives: the life we show people, and the life within. As we go down the rabbit hole with pornography, the distance between our public and private life expands.

We end up asking the question, who am I? Am I the good guy people see? Or am I the horny, sex-obsessed werewolf that comes out after everyone is asleep? Clicking, searching, hungry to devour breasts and butts. Enthralled by the novelty and endless options of the chase. Seeking the affirmation of pretty faces and willing eyes.

We know the shame that follows only brings emptiness. The rush of an orgasm is replaced with feelings of resignation and worthlessness, especially if we have tried to stop the behavior at some point. But what is the way out?

CHAPTER 1
BEING ALONE

THE FIRST TIME I SAW PORN, I WAS EIGHT years old. I was at a gas station with a mini-mart. While my grandmother was getting gas, I walked into the store. I went to the magazines near the front and saw a magazine that I didn't recognize. It was a little higher up. The name of the magazine escapes me, but the letters had vines wrapping between them. It was nature-themed with a cheeky reference to nakedness in the garden of Eden.

I grabbed it. On the first page I opened to, I saw an adult woman on a bed naked. It was exhilarating. I'd never seen anything like it. I quickly closed the magazine for fear that someone would catch me. In the next moment, my grandmother came in to pay.

Did she see me? I thought, panicked, still flushed with excitement.

When my friend Jay described his early discovery of porn, he said that "nobody had to tell me I had a secret." This was true for me. I now had a powerful secret.

I had always been intensely curious about girls' bodies. I have several memories of playing doctor or asking girls to show me their "penis." I didn't even know the word vagina. And the magazine planted this thought in my head: there must be more magazines like this where I could see every-thing. As soon as I saw it, I just wanted to see more. It didn't really go away. As I grew older, I felt the same draw, the same pull I had in that gas station. It was a deep desire.

When I got a little older, about twelve, I started looking for pornography. I found it in the neighbor's garbage. I found it at the office where I picked up the papers for my paper route. And when I couldn't find it, I began to steal it.

I had also figured out masturbation. Pairing porn with masturbation and orgasm cemented the habit. My searching and hunting now had this powerful purpose. It fed a growing hunger in me. It became my go-to escape from boredom, loneliness, and just about any other emotion in my life.

Pornography or masturbation was never talked about in my home. The one memory I have is when the subject of biker magazines with topless women came up at dinner. My dad was in sales and would call on the local Harley Davidson shop. I went with him one afternoon and had been caught paging through one of the magazines. On hearing this, my mom said to my dad in a shaming tone, "You never look at those magazines, do you?" I don't remember how he responded. But the message I got was there was only one acceptable answer to that question.

I tried to help myself. When I was fifteen years old, I bought a book at a church bookstore called *Eros Defiled* about sexuality. I tried to read the book and get some guidance, but it didn't really help. I still felt alone. I was still looking at porn. And I was feeling more and more guilty about it. I knew deep down this was out of alignment with my faith, but I still kept going to it.

Just after I turned eighteen, I moved into my first apartment. By then I also had a VCR. I could rent pornography. I had a roommate, but I didn't see him often. I do remember he had an old, recorded porno VHS he had forgotten about. I watched it so often, it broke. We never spoke of it.

No one knew what was going on with me. What made matters worse is that I had a second shift job at a print shop downtown. I was getting home at 2:00 a.m., jacked up from work, and I couldn't go to sleep till 4:00 a.m. I got in the habit of renting videos and buying magazines when I had the money.

About this time, I had started going to a commuter college and attending the Christian fellowship on campus. At one of the first meetings, a woman came in to speak from a ministry in town. She ran Christian support groups in the area of sexuality. In her talk, she spoke frankly about pornography and masturbation. She said both words out loud and mentioned that some of us might be trapped.

When she said it, it was like a light shined on me. It cut right to my core. All the hiding, all the places where I'd tried to be quiet and tried not to tell anybody. It felt like she was seeing right through me.

The fact that she just even said it in a talk validated me. I thought, *I'm not the only one.* I thought about trying to say something to her, but I was too ashamed to talk to her and I was already late for my job.

I had this naive thought that just hearing the truth from this speaker would somehow help me change—ideally without having to tell anybody.

But the next night, I was standing outside my apartment in a misty rain. It was two in the morning, and I had a ten-dollar bill in my hand. I was on the way to the train station to buy a porn magazine from the twenty-four-hour news stand, and I stopped in a moment of hesitation.

I remembered the speaker at school. I remembered how I'd felt alive as she was talking, as she explained the predicament I was in.

"Am I going to do this again?" I asked myself.

It was then I noticed I was standing next to a mailbox. Now, this was 1990, before email and Facebook. I suddenly had this thought: what if I went into my apartment and wrote a letter to the speaker? That's all I could think to do.

Then I had an even better idea. I'd put the ten dollars in the envelope with the letter, seal it, and mail it.

I ran back inside.

"I was going to use this ten dollars to buy porn tonight," my letter read. "But I'm putting it in this envelope to keep myself safe. And I'm mailing it to you."

I got her address from the phonebook and went right back to the mailbox. It was a small victory. I went to bed and didn't look at porn.

A couple of days later, I still hadn't looked at porn. I remember coming back from the grocery store with my roommate, and he pressed the answering machine button.

In the middle of the house, the voice of the speaker started playing. She had received my letter and left a message. She didn't say anything about the pornography or the masturbation, but she thanked me for writing her and told me sweetly that God loved me.

"Who is that?" my roommate asked.

I shrugged it off and told him I'd heard her speak last week at college.

Even though the answering machine message was embarrassing, I felt seen by her. I had finally told someone about my pornography use, and she wasn't judging me or condemning me.

That was the first time I reached out for help. Her reaction was so loving and caring.

Some thirty years later, you're reading this book. You put down your own money to buy it.

I want you to know you're seen by me. I understand where you're coming from. If you're struggling with porn, if you're struggling with masturbation, if you're in this endless spiral and you can't get free from it. I know what you're going through. And I know the shame that goes along with it. I get it. I'm here with you.

Maybe you have tried to tell someone in your life. Or maybe you are still trying to do this on your own. Either way, I want you to know this can be a scary step. But I want to encourage you.

You are not alone.

THE PRISON

C. S. Lewis writes, "After all, almost the main work of life is to come out of ourselves, out of the little, dark prison we are all born in."[1]

I have this memory as an eight-year-old, the same year I discovered pornography. I woke up in our house in rural Florida. It was a school day, but I was home sick.

I looked in the house for my mom and my little brother and sister. Calling out to them was no use. The station wagon was not in the long, dirt driveway.

I was a kid who could take care of myself. My mom probably didn't want to wake me. But something about being sick left me vulnerable to the feeling of being alone.

I started to cry uncontrollably.

The phone suddenly rang. I answered in tears. It was my grandfather from Milwaukee. Now, my grandfather was not a touchy-feely guy. But he knew something was wrong and asked where my mom was. As I told him what happened and why I was home alone, I started to calm down.

I don't remember what he said, but after the call I felt better. I turned on the TV and watched Mr. Rogers until my mom came home.

---

1. C. S. Lewis, *The Collected Letters of C. S. Lewis, Vol. 3* (New York: HarperSanFrancisco, 2007), 759.

I want to draw attention to how alone I felt in that moment. I was scared. I was crying uncontrollably. Even though I knew my mom would return, I felt abandoned. Deep down I think we all carry this fear of being alone. It's not just a fear of being alone in any given moment but also the idea that we are alone in life.

Thomas Merton writes that most men "are averse to being alone, or to feeling alone, that they do everything they can to forget their solitude."[2]

The older we get, the better we are at covering up and burying this feeling.

Think about yourself. How have you managed having that small, scared child deep within you? Have you tried to ignore it by distracting yourself? Have you avoided yourself? Have you tried to keep busy? Or maybe you have tried to numb the feeling, using powerful substances to medicate and take away the ache.

"By means of distraction," Thomas Merton writes. "A man can avoid his own company twenty-four hours a day."

This was me. The path I chose for many years was distraction and escape.

For many of us, there is no more intoxicating and thrilling escape than the pursuit of porn and

---

2. Thomas Merton, "Philosophy of Solitude," *Disputed Questions* (San Diego: Harvest Book, 1960), 178.

porn behaviors. It is always available. Its variety and sense of freedom provides endless fascination and surprise. In the fantasy, we are in complete control. We feel significant and powerful. It fills us temporarily with a sense of connection and intimacy. And it usually ends in an orgasm.

C. S. Lewis warned of a danger that comes with this chase. It leads to us back into the prison of ourself—increasingly cut off from others and from reality.

"The danger," he writes, "is that of coming to love the prison."[3]

The good news is the path you have chosen by picking up this book leads to freedom. And I will help you get there.

When I was at the beginning of this journey, I loved this quote by G. K. Chesterton: "Anything worth doing is worth doing badly."[4]

That concept was freeing to me. Struggling on this journey is worth it, and it's worth looking bad. Don't be afraid to be messy.

If you're like me, you have had (or will have) a lot of starts and stops before you really get this. Don't

---

3. C. S. Lewis, *The Collected Letters of C. S. Lewis, Vol. 3* (New York: HarperSanFrancisco, 2007), 759.

4. Adapted from the original G. K. Chesterton quote, "If a thing is worth doing, it is worth doing badly"; G. K. Chesterton, "Folly and Female Education," *What's Wrong with the World* (London: Cassell, 1910), 320.

give in to the lie that if you can't do this perfectly, you can't do it at all.

You can't do this perfectly. But you *can* do this.

After years of working on a program and getting some freedom for myself, I started a group to help others. At the group, I would share different stories from my life. One night, I told that story about the ten dollars.

At the end of the group, one of the men came up to me and said he really appreciated that story. Then, out of his wallet, he pulled a single ten-dollar bill. He said when he came to group that night, he knew in the back of his mind he had ten dollars. He asked if I could put this in the offering bucket of my church. He simply said, "I was going to act out tonight with this ten dollars, but I need to stay safe, and I need to give it to you."

As you start to get freedom, as you start to be vulnerable with others and tell people your story, you get an opportunity to help others.

I am giving you permission to be vulnerable and make mistakes. This is worth doing.

CHAPTER 2

THE PORN SOLUTION

"WHY DID YOU REACH OUT TO ME?" I ASKED.

I start every call like this with guys who are interested in working with me as a coach. I'll never forget the answer from one young man.

"I need you to teach me how to hate porn," he said matter-of-factly.

I had never heard this response before. "Tell me more."

"I feel so bad about myself when I look at porn. I feel weak and ashamed. Whatever I do, I can't seem to stop. I've gone two months before but have never gone longer. I'm lying to my fiancée. I don't know what to do . . . I need to hate it."

I get his logic. If we hate something, it would be easier to quit.

"Do you like Dr. Pepper?" I asked.

"Uh, sure," he answered.

"Well, I love Dr. Pepper," I said. "It's one of my favorite drinks. But it doesn't work with my health and weight-loss goals. I also have a hard time drinking just one. So it's not part of my life anymore.

"Do you think that my taste has changed?" I asked. "Do you think I woke up one day and started to hate the taste of Dr. Pepper?

"I guarantee that if you opened a cold Dr. Pepper right now and made me drink it, I would still love the taste."

Before we go any further, I need to share something vital. It's completely shifted my thinking in recovery.

We see, over and over, porn as a problem that needs to be solved.

It's called an epidemic. It's called a crisis. There's plenty of articles about it being bad for your brain. It's a reported cause of erectile dysfunction, "brain fog," and divorces. It leads to sex trafficking and exploitation. It demeans women. Reportedly it causes depression and anxiety. It's a new drug, more powerful than heroin, which makes us all addicts.

If we look for help at church or at our house of worship, our porn usage is often treated as a battle for purity. Porn is our cunning enemy entrapping us in lust and virtual adultery. Using porn shows a fundamental lack of self-control. It's a sign that we lack spiritual discipline in the face of temptation. A weakness of our "flesh."

Some of those things may be true, but when you're struggling to go porn free, these messages make you feel three things.

ASHAMED

Why would anyone knowingly get addicted to this? Why would anyone participate in demeaning women or sex trafficking? Why would anyone choose this over a healthy marriage?

"Guilt, of course, is feeling bad about one's actions," writes Fr. Gregory Boyle. "But shame is feeling bad about oneself. Failure, embarrassment, weakness, overwhelming worthlessness, and feeling disgracefully 'less than'—all permeating the marrow of the soul."[1]

We buy into this. We believe we are not good enough—broken. One of the guys I worked with concluded he was "disgusting" at his core. That's shame talking.

---

1. Gregory Boyle, *Tattoos on the Heart* (New York: Free Press, 2010), 46.

HELPLESS

What can we do about it? Porn is powerful and pervasive. It's accessible everywhere and more stimulating than ever. We are the unwilling victim. Once it gets its hook in us, we're rendered powerless. We're trapped. We keep coming back and back for more and more. Our brain has been rewired and hijacked.

HOPELESS

Change is impossible. A quick review of porn usage online, and it's obvious that we're not alone. At any given time, three or four porn sites are in the top ten for most visits in the world.

The comedian Chris Rock shared about his porn addiction in a recent Netflix special. The audience laughed somewhat awkwardly after his admission. "I know," he joked. "Billion-dollar industry, just me, right?"[2]

We have a sense that everyone does this, and yet we're the only ones who are struggling. We're in an ocean drowning with no shore in sight. It's overwhelming.

Treating porn as a problem makes us feel ashamed, helpless, and hopeless. These feelings

---

2. Chris Rock, *Chris Rock: Tamborine* (Netflix, 2018).

work against us, though. They keep us stuck and make going porn free impossible.

PORN IS NOT THE PROBLEM FOR US. IT'S THE SOLUTION.

When we go to porn, we're escaping, we're numbing, we're looking for excitement, we're looking for enjoyment. It's an elusive sensation.

We're not going because we want to feel bad about ourselves. We're going to feel good.

Remember the first time seeing it? There was a thrill, an excitement. Sure, it felt like a secret. Maybe we were ashamed a little bit, but mostly it felt good.

Porn is a powerful solution to a variety of problems. It's on-demand 24/7. There are endless searches you can do and endless novelty to fascinate us. It's perfectly designed to give us exactly what we want. It's enjoyable to us. We like the taste, even better than Dr. Pepper.

This may be a hard truth if we believe that it's a sin based on our faith. Or that it is addicting based on research that we've read. Or that it hurts our wife deeply. We may be conflicted about the consequences, but no doubt, whether consciously or not, it's still a solution.

In our first attempts at recovery, we try to control porn and porn behaviors. It could be with a resolution like, "I will never do this again." It could be installing a filter or app blocker. It could be giving up a device like a phone or laptop. I once let my neighbors borrow my VCR indefinitely because I couldn't stop renting porn.

But if that's all we do, we're in trouble.

In the early twentieth century, a group of moralists and politicians prohibited alcohol sales and manufacturing in America. It was called the Great Prohibition. It seemed like a good idea at the time.

But what did it do? It just made a whole bunch of bootleggers and "rum-runners" out of alcohol drinkers. People were making gin in their bathtubs. My hometown of Chicago is notorious for being the home of speakeasies and mobsters that rebelled against prohibition.

Incidentally, Russia tried it again in the 1980s. Gorbachev outlawed alcohol, and it led to a sugar shortage because so many people were trying to make their own booze.

The problem with prohibition is it made alcohol the problem. But it failed to solve the problem of alcoholism or why people were using alcohol.

We do the same thing. When we make porn the problem, we try to fix it using one tool or another. We think if we just find the right filter or an accountability partner, then we will do the right thing.

We think if we educate ourselves about it, read articles and Reddit posts, that will create change. We assume that if we get the right type of thinking, we'll make the right choices. As Jason George from the GRIZ podcast, often says, "Information alone does not lead to transformation."[3]

If the underlying problems are still there, we'll continue to evade any safeguards or fixes we install. We'll lie to our accountability partners. We'll circumvent our knowledge or ignore it altogether. We're like bootleggers. We'll find a way.

When we make porn the problem, it distracts us from our real needs, or, worse, it makes our needs the enemy. This consequence is the real tragedy of our predicament.

This fact is particularly true with guys from a faith background. We're taught that porn is lust. It is a battleground for purity and obedience. But underneath we have these powerful needs driving our behaviors. We desire things like love, connection, significance, intimacy, and touch. All good things.

But all too often in our attempts to "hate porn," we end up hating our legitimate needs.

This mistake is made over and over in church groups. Guys pretend to have it together or hide behind scripture and false spirituality. If they

3. Greg Ogden, *Transforming Discipleship* (United States: InterVarsity Press, 2016), 46.

didn't look at porn one week, they are filled with pride. If they looked at porn, they are defeated and downcast. Dejected and crushed. Confused by their sudden fall.

When we're able to look at porn as a solution, we're able to look at needs in a healthier way. We can focus on the real problems.

I have used the word *recovery* a few times so far. Here's a definition: recovery is the process of getting healthy. It's an emotional, spiritual, and physical process.

There is no "magic bullet" quick fix. Recovery takes time. It is rooted in building skills and consistency over time to overcome challenges. It requires connection and commitment. In recovery, we overhaul our habits.

We put a spotlight on the emotional triggers that drive our behaviors. *What are the real needs?* We expose mistaken beliefs and lies that we are tempted to believe in order to stay in our habit with porn. *What lies am I believing that make me feel ashamed, helpless, and hopeless?*

We eliminate the places in our life that make it easy to go to porn. There is wisdom to creating obstacles to pornography. We don't have to make it easy to get to porn. I think of the alcoholic who's recovering from alcohol. He doesn't keep a whole bunch of beer in his fridge to test himself. But that isn't the whole answer, not when there's a bar down the street. In the same way, filters and accountability partners aren't enough.

When we make porn the problem, we ignore our real needs. We'll come back to talking about our needs, but first let's talk about the costs of using porn and the reasons why it is a poor solution for us.

CHAPTER 3

BUT WAIT, ISN'T PORN AN ADDICTION?

I USE THE WORD *ADDICTION* **RARELY IN** this book. Compulsive pornography use with masturbation is not considered an addiction by many. Sex-positive experts say that the word *addiction* shames genuine sexual curiosity or hypersexuality. They are also quick to point out that pornography addiction is not a diagnosis recognized by the Diagnostic and Statistical Manual of Mental Disorders, 5th Edition (DSM-5), the bible for mental health professionals.

On the other end of the spectrum, conservative religious types also push back on the word *addiction* because it seems to justify a lack of self-control. It's seen as an excuse for repeating sin. It also can be in conflict with theology about being a new creation or saved.

The word *addict* is also problematic. I avoid using it for a different reason. It neither motivates nor encourages a recovering person. And as we recover, it becomes increasingly inaccurate.

For the purposes of getting porn free, it is helpful to view all addiction as a habit.

"Addiction, in its varying degrees, is an extreme version of a habit," writes Dr. A. Thomas Horvath. "And overcoming addiction occurs using the same processes we use to change habits."[1]

This may be hard to see at first. Compulsive behavior can seem automatic. Like it's wired in us. We feel we don't have a choice. For an example, when I ask guys about emotional triggers that lead to porn use, the first one most mentioned is almost always "being alone."

At first, I assumed it was the fear of being alone that was a trigger, especially since I struggled with that. When I was alone, I felt anxious or unlovable. For me, the emotional trigger was in those feelings. But many guys who would consider themselves introverts said they didn't fear being alone. They liked it.

---

1. Dr. A. Thomas Horvath, *Sex, Drugs, Gambling, and Chocolate: A Workbook for Overcoming Addictions* (Atascadero, CA: Impact Publishers, 2003), 1.

Being alone was a trigger of opportunity. They had associated it with porn. Every time they were alone, they would use porn. It was automatic, like Pavlov's dog salivating when the bell rang. But as powerful as that association is, it is still, at its core, a habit.

We have lots of automatic habits in our life. Brushing our teeth in the morning. Drinking coffee. Watching TV after work. Speeding on the highway.

What distinguishes an addiction from common habits then? Excessive costs.

It's simple. Horvath summarizes that involvement with anything has a cost, and the cost is usually proportional to the benefits we receive. Think of it as the value or our satisfaction. If we get great benefit out of doing something that has a low cost, we're thrilled. Imagine being in the supermarket and your favorite ice cream was on sale for $1 per gallon. You would load up your cart.

But what if that same gallon was marked $10 or $20? We would feel ripped off or price gouged. What if we felt compelled to continue to buy it anyway? Addiction is like buying the outrageously expensive ice cream over and over. It's a rip off.

One challenge we face at the beginning of the recovery is we can be blind to the excessive costs of compulsive pornography use.

"The cost of a thing is the amount of what I will call life which is required to be exchanged for it, immediately or in the long run."

—Cal Newport[2]

The first question I ask my coaching clients is, "What has porn cost you?" Despite coming to me for help with recovery, guys surprisingly have trouble answering at first. But as we dig in together, two costs come up over and over: the cost of time, and the cost of living a divided life.

THE COST OF TIME

"Matt, porn is costing me time." When I ask guys what porn cost them, that's usually the first answer they come up with.

"Tell me more about time," I say. "Why is time the thing that's getting you to apply for coaching? Why is time the thing that's preeminently on your mind when you think about what porn has cost you?"

"Well, I feel like I could be more productive," they reply, "if I didn't have porn in my life. Just the hours wasted looking at porn and searching. It feels like it's a bad use of time."

---

2. Henry David Thoreau, as quoted by Cal Newport, *Digital Minimalism: Choosing a Focused Life in a Noisy World* (New York: Portfolio/Penguin,2019), 39.

Now there's lots of things we do that are bad uses of our time. We watch TV, we watch too much sports, we play video games. We do a whole bunch of things that maybe aren't the best uses of our time, but we don't hire a life coach to help us figure out how to watch less TV, right?

But porn is different for you. That's why you're reading this book.

Dr. Doug Weiss is a psychologist in Colorado who specializes in sex addiction. He has an exercise he does with new clients. He has a guy come up with his dollar value per hour. How much do you make a year, divided by the hours in the work week? Maybe it's $80 an hour.

Then he asks the guy to estimate how much porn he looks at. Let's say it's three or four hours a week. Do the math. That's $16,000 a year of lost productivity time on porn. The thought is that we work for a certain dollar amount, so spending time with porn is kind of the equivalent of spending that money.

I get that there's opportunity cost in porn, but again, we could do lots of things with time. You could be refinishing a boat in your garage, and it could take a ton of time. It wouldn't even be worth the amount you could sell the boat for considering how much time you've put into it. Does that make it a bad use of time?

Is it *really* the hours spent that make it bad?

Ask yourself, what's underneath that? What does it mean to spend valuable time on something you don't want in your life? What's the true cost?

There are four main ways I've found that porn robs us of our time.

1. PORN DISHONORS OUR VALUE

It's something we don't want to do. Every time we go to it, it crushes us. It shakes our confidence. It makes us doubt our ability to make good choices and to follow through.

There are all sorts of internal consequences when we continually go back to something that we've sworn to stop. Every time we retreat into porn, it dishonors us.

Let's go back to the idea of building a boat in your garage. It could honor something about you. Maybe you're creative. Maybe you're good using your hands. Maybe there's something that comes alive when you are sanding. Maybe your dad and you used to work on projects together. There's a piece of you that comes alive when you're in your garage working on the boat. The hours spent honor the true self. They honor you.

Now there are things we do with our time that aren't quite as honoring. Video games are often thrown in this category. And there might come a point where that starts to dishonor your value, but we need fun things in our life, things that capture our interest—sports, leisure activities, etc. We need to have boundaries with them, but if we spend some time watching a game and it makes us feel good, and we're hanging with our friends, it doesn't dishonor us.

We're not waking up the next day going, "Oh, did I watch the Cubs game last night? All nine innings? Did I do that?"

I don't know anyone who wakes up the next morning and says, "Did I watch American Ninja Warrior again last night?"

"Hey, Bob, I gotta check in with you. I did it last night. I watched *American Ninja Warrior.* I watched for two hours. I even watched the bonus runs on YouTube. That's how bad it was. I binged on Ninja Warrior."

That conversation never happens.

When we press into activities that honor our true self, we come alive.

You might be a guitarist. It takes a lot of time to learn a Van Halen song. It takes literally hours, but if that's how you come alive, it honors you. It's a good use of your time.

If you've identified porn as an issue, a struggle, a place you don't want to go back to, then you're agreeing with me that it's dishonoring you, that it actually dishonors your personhood. It's not just your time, but it's your own value that it costs you. That's number one. It dishonors your time, but more importantly, it also dishonors your value.

2. PORN SPONTANEOUSLY OVERRIDES YOUR LIFE

Have you ever been up late, and you really should be going to bed, and next thing you know you're binging on porn for several hours? It totally overrode what you were going to do with your night. Have you ever had a project due, and you have to get some hours in it this week, but the next thing you know you're watching two or three hours of porn? It just takes over. You have time allotted to work on something—boom, all of a sudden you're in porn. It also creates a lack of focus. You should be focusing on something during your workday, but now you're thinking about porn. Is it becoming obsessive thinking? Are you thinking about the next time you can act out?

It's never planned. You could have ten minutes free while your wife's in the shower—and, boom, you're on your phone. It overrode whatever you were doing because you saw an opportunity. Guys are always talking about staying up late. I've even heard of guys waking up early in the morning before the kids, and all of a sudden they're doing a search.

This is part of what people mean when they say that porn is taking time from them. It spontaneously overrides your life. We feel out of control. We feel like things are unmanageable. We feel powerless. There's a big consequence to that override. Have you ever been in a conversation with someone who constantly interrupts you? That's what porn is doing—it's constantly interrupting our life.

3. PORN RUINS THE NEXT DAY

Acting out today has a time effect tomorrow too. If you stay up late tonight and feel like crap the next day and get up later, you start spilling over. If you binge for a weekend, it can screw up your entire week. If you don't get stuff done, if you procrastinate, all the things you put on hold that you didn't want to deal with come flooding back to you.

After a tough loss in college football, you might hear a coach say, "Don't let Ohio State beat you twice." It means that it's very easy to let the sinking feeling of a loss carry over to the next week.

The next day, even if we're not looking at porn, it's beating us, because we're feeling like crap. And the porn hangover can last for days. It's not just those hours that you were binging, but it's all the cascade of consequences in the days to follow.

4. PORN ROBS YOU OF YOUR PRESENCE

Here's the fourth thing that it does with your time. It robs you of your presence. When you're acting out with porn and hiding in your office, or your bedroom, or wherever you go to look at porn, you're physically removing yourself from other people's presence. I've heard of guys who have kids and retreat into their basement or their offices when their kids are in the house to look at porn. Just the act of going to the office or withdrawing robs children of their father's presence.

Even when you're there, you can be distracted by the porn, thinking about when you can act out again. If you're waiting for your wife to go to sleep so you can get up and go look at porn, it's not a particularly loving and honoring way of being in her presence. Believe me; I've done this. When you're sitting around in the presence of others and you're thinking about how you can get out of this so you can act out, you're ignoring the reality that's in front of you, and the love that's in front of you, and the relationship that's in front of you.

You're not present even when you're there because porn is in your head and you're continuing to think about it. That's where time comes in—this is what guys mean when they say it robs them of their time. It's about your value, it's about your schedule, it's about how you order your life, and it's about your presence.

Here's the thing: if we wave a magic wand right now and porn's not a part of your life, you're still going to waste time. You're not going to be the most productive guy in the world just because you have all these extra hours. Your hours will be taken up by other things. But if we waved a magic wand and eliminated porn from your life, there's more potential that the activities that fill the space could honor your true self and could really fill more needs in your life.

THE COST OF LIVING A DIVIDED LIFE

I always recommend guys take ownership in recovery by developing a WHY. It summarizes the thing that they are most sick and tired of in addiction and what they are moving toward in recovery.

My WHY is this:

I'm sick and tired of agreeing with the lie that I'm unlovable, and I want to be the same on the inside as on the outside.

I'll share more later on how I developed this WHY and how to develop your own, but for now, focus on what I want most in recovery.

"To be the same on the inside as on the outside."
To me, that means wholeness and integration.

The Cloven Viscount is a dark tale about a viscount named Medardo.[3] A viscount is like a nobleman who has a castle and an area of land and people who support him. The story opens as the young nobleman goes to war. He joins a battle against the Turks.

He's inexperienced when he goes to his first day of battle. Almost immediately, he is separated from his horse, which is not a good sign. But he's emboldened by the fighting, and he charges a cannon on foot. The cannon is fired, and he takes a direct shot, which cuts him completely in half.

Later in the day, they have a truce where the enemies could go around and collect their dead and their wounded. Half of the nobleman is found alive. After hours of surgery, they stitch him up and send him home.

When he gets home, he locks himself up in his room for several days. When he emerges, he starts doing some very strange things. The man who came back to the castle is mean and brutal. He starts a reign of terror.

He's the judge in the town, and he starts harshly sentencing men to torture or to death. There are

3. Italo Calvino, *The Nonexistent Knight & the Cloven Viscount* (New York: Harcourt Brace Jovanovich, 1977).

people who owe him money, and he's merciless about collecting it or killing them. Just being an evil dictator isn't good enough for him. He actually starts terrorizing people, firebombing houses, and lighting fires. Also, he carries a sharp sickle-like knife, and he will cut fruit orchards in half. At one point, he bisects all the apples in an apple orchard.

He is resentful, unjust, vengeful—he is complete evil. He has no empathy, and he's just driven by power. The town and the people in his kingdom are completely scared of him.

It turns out that in the fateful battle, the other half of Medardo lived, too.

The other half is found by two hermits lying under some of the corpses on the battlefield. The hermits are wise with using herbal remedies and little concoctions, which save him. This half is completely virtuous. As he makes his way throughout Europe, he does good deeds and is completely kind to everyone in his path. Eventually, he makes it back to the kingdom.

So both halves of the men are back and operating in their natures. The one half, Gramo (the Bad), is terrorizing people and doing horrible things. The kind and virtuous half, Buono (the Good), is taking care of people and animals who have been hurt by his other half.

Then both halves of the man fall in love with the same peasant woman, Pamela. Gramo sees her and wants to possess her. He wants to take her up into the castle and lock her in a tower. He's driven, and he convinces her father to let him marry her. Buono falls in love with Pamela in the woods, where they cultivate a relationship. He desires to be with her, too, but does not have the same drive as his evil half. This frustrates Pamela.

"I'm beginning to realize that you're a bit too soft," she says. "Instead of attacking that other half of yours for all the swinish things he does, you seem almost to pity him."

"Of course I do," replies Buono. "I know what it means to be half a man."[4]

Buono is virtuous and exceedingly kind, but he is passive. The townspeople also get annoyed with Buono because he avoids confrontation with Gramo. His good actions do not solve the problems created by Gramo. What's worse is that he preaches to them a lot and is always moralizing and telling them what to do.

The story ends with an epic conclusion where the two rivals end up fighting in a duel. Here's what's unexpected. They're unable to hurt one another because they're both incomplete.

"Certainly if instead of half duelers there had been two whole ones, they would have wounded each other again and again," the narrator says.

---

4. Calvino, *The Nonexistent Knight & the Cloven Viscount*, 216.

"Gramo fought with fury and veracity, yet never managed to launch his attacks, just where his enemy was; Buono had correct mastery, but never did more than pierce the Viscount's cloak."[5]

During their fight, the one-legged men become unbalanced. They fall into one another, and their bodies entangle. The town doctor takes advantage of this opportunity and sews them together. The two halves are integrated into a whole man. It's a happy ending.

Think about your story. What if the part of you that comes alive in porn and the good guy you show people were split into two men?

Would either half be complete?

We often assume that the virtuous part of us, the good guy we show people, is who we really are. We think recovery is about eliminating the porn guy in us.

But we are invested in living this way. We like being able to be selfish and narcissistic, but showing people a good and humble guy on the outside.

But recovery is about wholeness.

In the story, we see these two halves fighting for the hand of Pamela, each one counteracting one another. When Gramo decides to pursue Pamela, it's because he sees love is important, yet has no capacity to love. He is driven by his passion

---

5. Calvino, *The Nonexistent Knight & the Cloven Viscount*, 243.

to possess her, yet he has no empathy. He doesn't care for others; he only thinks of himself.

However, Buono is also incomplete. He is kind and always thinking the best of people. But he is gullible. He's taken advantage of several times. At one point, he gives his crutch to a man who claims to be lame, but the man was pretending. He took the crutch home and beat his wife with it. Buono is also passive. When Pamela comes to him and says that she wants to marry him, he insists she marry Gramo.

In some ways, Pamela is like our wife saying, "Why won't you fight for me? Why won't you do what you need to do?"

But Buono doesn't have the capacity by himself. He's incomplete.

WHOLENESS IS THE GOAL OF OUR RECOVERY

When I say I want to be the same on the inside as on the outside, what I'm really getting at is that we need to integrate the parts of us that have been hidden and that came alive in porn with our outside self. When we're using porn, there is drive, and energy, and excitement. We need that type of energy, commitment, and drive in our life.

Obviously, we want to eliminate the behaviors, but we don't want to eliminate the needs or the passion. Otherwise, we end up a passive good guy who can't do what needs to be done.

In *Self-Discipline in 10 Days*, Theodore Bryant uses the classic story of Dr. Jekyll and Mr. Hyde to illustrate a similar point. "Think of that part of you that wants self-discipline as Dr. Jekyll," Bryant writes, "and the part of you that fights your attempts at self-discipline as Hyde."[6]

We all have this rebellious side that doesn't want to be told what to do. But Bryant invites us to consider our approach. He writes:

> "Do not however think of your Hyde side as an enemy. Think, instead, of Hyde as the part of you that is creative, fun-loving, and pleasure-seeking; the child side of yourself. You do not want to do battle with Hyde, but you want to recruit Hyde as a partner who supports your self-discipline efforts."[7]

We need fun and excitement in our recovery. Ultimately, we can never win if we're just trying to eliminate the part of us that emerges in porn. We're that guy too. We're competitive and driven. We're passionate. We're playful. We seek variety and

---

6. Theodore Bryant, *Self-Discipline in 10 Days* (Seattle, WA: Hub Publishing, 2011), 8.
7. Bryant, *Self-Discipline in 10 Days*, 8.

adventure. These are good things, and we're incomplete without them.

CHAPTER 4

EITHER WE GET CAUGHT OR WE GET COURAGE

A LOT OF US START THIS JOURNEY WITH one of two things happening: either we get caught by someone important in our life, or we get courage and we start talking about what's really going on. We start being honest about our struggle.

No matter how you begin, the next step is the same.

It was two years into my marriage. It was a hot June night, and my wife, Janice, and I had spent all weekend at church. There was this famous worship leader visiting. Maybe you've heard of him—Matt Redman. He's written a whole bunch of famous worship songs. He came into town with a pastor from the UK, and they did a conference at my church, and it was amazing. People came from out of town for this. When we left, everyone was encouraged; everyone was on a spiritual high.

We got home on a Saturday night after the conference, and Janice went to bed early, at ten o'clock.

Back then, just being left alone was the opportunity trigger to look at porn. When I was confident that she was asleep, I slipped down the hall to my home office.

I logged onto the computer. Back then, the computer took a little more time to set up and dial in, but soon I was clicking through some of my favorite sites, looking at pictures, downloading things, and I lost track of time.

It was the early days of the internet. But even then there was a seemingly endless supply of rabbit holes to go down. I found a gold mine in newsgroups (a precursor to various internet forums like Reddit). In minutes, I could read sex stories, click through fetish categories, and view uploaded pictures and video clips. It was the Wild West.

I loved the hunt. When I would get an idea in my head, I would obsessively chase it until I found just what I was looking for. My computer provided me with endless variety and novelty. The search to me was as thrilling as the orgasm that followed.

That night, I was in a complete tunnel vision state where I lost track of time. I had no idea how much had elapsed when I heard Janice's voice. "What are you doing?"

She stood at the doorway of our home office waiting for an answer as I scrambled to turn off the monitor and pull up my boxer shorts. She had opened the door, and I was caught red-handed. There was no cover-up. No minimizing. No talking my way out of this. In that moment, the secret I had been hiding for most of my life was totally exposed.

I had shared with her about my struggle with pornography when we were dating, but I made it sound like it was twenty years in the past. I was not honest about how hard it was or that it was still a challenge. I tried to do it on my own. I'd resolve to not use porn for periods, get rid of my computer, or loan my VCR to neighbors. I would do these things to try to block myself from using, but I'd always go back to it somehow. It would end up in that shame cycle where I swore off ever doing it again. Then I'd do it again and feel horrible.

Janice asked a lot of hard questions that first night and in the nights to follow.

I remember trying to explain myself, but even I didn't know why I was doing this. I never felt good about it. I had tried to stop but I always went back.

That night, two things were true. First, I was desperate to try fix things. I wanted things to go back to normal. I wished that she hadn't woken up. I was desperate to not feel the shame and guilt.

But at the same time, I felt a rush of freedom. It's the same feeling you have when you get fired from a job you don't like. You're scared about what's next, but you're happy you never have to work there again.

My secret porn life was now out in the open—for better or for worse.

We forget that there's a burden to hiding. There's a burden to carrying around that feeling of shame we have when we continually act out and hide it from the people we love.

Before we went to sleep that night, Janice said something to me I will always remember. "This is not about me," she said. "But you need help."

God gave her wisdom and grace in this moment. She knew this was bigger than her. For many people struggling with porn, their partners think it's a rejection of them specifically. I totally get that. It is betrayal of trust and affection.

But most of us discovered porn as kids and have been struggling ever since. Long before we ever met our wives, this was a problem. If we had the tools or willpower to stop, we would have.

My recovery story started with getting caught, and I know that's true for a lot of guys. I remember one story about a guy who had been looking at porn on his phone before jumping in his car with his significant other. You know how Bluetooth connects to your phone and plays whatever was playing last?

All of a sudden, the sounds of two people having sex filled the car. That was a tough conversation.

But I've also heard plenty of stories of brave guys who were sick and tired of their double life, who took the step of talking to their wife or a close friend.

My podcast, Porn Free Radio, started with episode one about coming clean, and it was about breaking through the shame, breaking through the isolation, and taking a step into exposure—and into being known.

To be free, we need this exposure. I have seldom heard of successful recovery in secret. So why do we avoid it? There are three reasons.

LOOKING BAD

Deep down, we don't want to look bad. We want to look like we're competent. In the first year of marriage, my wife referred to me as "the strong one." I was invested in this image. I avoided looking bad at all costs. But under the surface, I had internalized that I was not good enough and unlovable.

If we already struggle with that feeling, looking bad intensifies the shame we already feel. We don't want to expose our weakness. We don't want to expose sin. We don't want to expose things we've done that we're not proud of. Because if we were to expose that, we believe the lie that the person we reveal our weakness to would reject us. We're invested in not being rejected, especially if we're walking around with a wound that says we're unlovable. We're constantly trying to prove externally that we're good enough, and we go to extraordinary lengths to look like a good guy.

LOSS AVERSION

The second reason is a little more complicated. It's tied in with the theory of loss aversion. Have you ever heard of loss aversion? Studies about what motivates people have found that people are much more motivated by the fear of loss than they are by what they might gain.

We lose more satisfaction in a loss than we gain in a win.

Say you got $100 off the retail price of a set of tires for your car. You shopped around and know you got a good deal. You saved $100! You're happy.

But on the way home, you drove ten miles over the limit and got a $100 speeding ticket. Bummer! You lost $100.

The amount was the same, but which feeling would you remember more?

If it were me, the speeding ticket would ruin my day. I would fixate on it. The loss is a more powerful feeling than a gain.

That's why limited-time offers work in marketing. We fear losing the savings. It's also why I will drive across town to avoid a seventy-five cent library fine, but forget to bring my five-dollar off coupon to the grocery store.

But what does this have to do with quitting porn?

The gain that we receive from getting free of this, from living in freedom, is not as motivating to us as the fear of losing the comfort of porn.

Many of us discovered porn at an early age, and it became a primary way to deal with powerful emotions, like sadness, anger, resentment, fear, or even anxiety. A part of us is wholly invested in using porn and doesn't want to give it up.

The fear of loss is much more powerful than what we might gain in freedom. Taking away this thing feels so much more painful than an abstract potential gain.

Even if we examine how this is costing us, there's still a part of us that says, "No, I don't want to let go. It's the way I get comfort. When I've had a hard day, this is the way I get release. I don't want to lose that. I don't want to be penalized."

FEAR OF PAIN

This brings us to our last reason, fear of pain. Why do we escape to porn? Why do we numb with porn? Why do we procrastinate with porn? What are we avoiding?

We are avoiding pain, and we hate pain. Ed Sheeran has a song called "Pain Eraser." It's about alcohol, but for us, porn is our pain eraser. To be exposed to someone we love, to be honest about how this is dominating our thoughts, would require us to move out of this place of hiddenness.

And what's that going to bring? It's going to bring pain. One guy I talked to called porn the salve, like it was this healing salve you could rub into a wound to make it feel better. Our fear is that if we're exposed, then we'll have to feel all that pain, and we avoid that.

We don't want to lose those things. That's one of the reasons that even after we're caught, we continue to lie and hide.

Another way we avoid pain is by minimizing. That's one of the ways I did it. Early in recovery, my wife would come home and she said, "Did you look at anything inappropriate tonight? Did you cross any of your boundaries?" I would always answer no. It didn't matter if I looked or didn't look; the fear of exposure and the pain I thought would follow was so great that I would lie. I was still facing the problem of not wanting to look bad, not wanting to lose this go-to solution, not wanting to feel pain, that I would say, "No, nothing's wrong. I didn't look at anything."

Exposure is necessary because it is the first step to being known. Being known is scary at first, but it's the place where we will get free. See, in our desperation to hide our porn life, to cover our tracks, to look good . . . we hide our needs, our pain, and our wounds. This leaves us alone and hurting.

But there is good news. There are three gifts of being known.

NO MORE HIDING

We don't realize how much energy it takes to hide sneaking off to porn. Keeping up the false front, showing "the good guy" to the people in our life, then retreating to our secret life when we're alone.

Imagine a guy who is married to two wives and has two families, and he's constantly going back and forth and constantly trying to hide his bigamy. That's what we're doing. We go back and forth, back and forth, between these two worlds.

Hiding takes an incredible toll, not to mention all the mental strain of the shame. When we hide, we feel all sorts of things. We feel a lack of confidence because we can't quit. We feel like a hypocrite because we're not living in alignment with our values. I've had guys tell me that the main thing getting them into recovery is not because they feel bad at looking at porn—they like looking at porn—but they can't stand the fact that they keep lying to their wives. Lying is taking a toll. Deep down, we know the truth and every day we have to suppress it. It eats us from the inside out.

WE CAN FOCUS ON THE REAL PROBLEM

The second gift is we can focus on the real problem. Like we talked about earlier, the biggest problem that guys have when they first get into recovery is they treat porn like the problem. It's seen as a crisis. An epidemic. A battle. A betrayal.

Porn is the enemy. Porn is the problem.

But when you're hiding and avoiding pain—porn is the solution. We're not happy about it, but the problem for us is pain. It's the fear, it's the anxiety, it's the resentment, it's the boredom, it's the sadness, it's the depression, it's the entitlement. That's what we are escaping. That's what's driving the behavior. Porn is our solution.

When we are known, we can focus on the real problem. We can start to look for ways to meet those needs. How can I get more security in my life if I'm feeling fear? What can I do with the resentment and entitlement I feel? How can I affirm those parts of me that feel unlovable or rejected? What can I do when I'm bored? If we're constantly running and escaping, numbing, using the salve of porn, we never see the real places of pain in our life.

LOVE AND ACCEPTANCE

The third benefit of being known is we have the opportunity to experience love and acceptance. Nothing gets in when you're hiding. You want to know why? Because if someone sees the persona, you're putting out there, no matter how loving or accepting they are of that guy, deep down you're going to say, "Yeah, but they don't know the real me."

When my inside doesn't match my outside and someone gives me a compliment, it rolls right off my back. I can't receive it because no matter how good the compliment, it's counteracted by my secret. Internally, I believe the lie that I'm not good enough and if they knew the real me, they would reject me.

Being known, even in hard conversations with my wife about pornography, is where I first experienced her acceptance and love. When she said, "This isn't about me, but you need help," I heard the empathy and the care. She was saying to me, "You have a real problem. This is hurting you. I see it and you need help."

Now let's say that I was hiding that night and she didn't catch me, and we just talked generally about life. Would I feel known? Would I feel seen? No. I would be so entrenched in hiding and that no matter what she said to me, no matter how loving or caring she was, I wouldn't be able to receive it.

If you've been caught, but you realize you're still avoiding exposure, you're avoiding looking bad, you don't want to lose your go-to solution, or you're fearing pain, I want to encourage you to get current with the people in your life you've shared this with.

What do I mean by getting current? Telling them what's up. When was the last time you acted out? What are ways you're hiding? What are ways you're minimizing? What are some of the true threats in your life right now? Are there some habits that you've created around certain apps, websites, or times of the day? Get current. You've already had some exposure, so that means that you've opened yourself up to this. Go all the way. Be fully open.

If you haven't been caught yet, you need to find a place to start being honest. It may mean a hard conversation with your wife or roommate. It may mean joining a group or trusting a close friend. It may mean getting a counselor or coach.

But you need to tell the whole story to someone because it's going to lead to relief.

Guys show up to the coaching groups I run and share their story, and they realize, "Man, this is a place I'm not hiding. One hour a week, I am not hiding. I want to get all the hours of my week to be not hiding, but I'm going to start with one."

In our groups, we can check in about the real problems. We start with sharing feelings, not a porn report. What are some of the powerful feelings coming up this week? Shame, stress, anger, boredom, fear. Those are the problems we need help navigating.

Love and acceptance from other guys who've been there can be healing. "Every man needs help," my friend and author Nate Larkin says. "And every man has some help to give."[1]

That's one of the powerful things about being in a group. It gives you a chance to practice vulnerability, you get a chance to practice honesty, and you get a chance to practice connection and acceptance.

---

1. Adapted from the original Nate Larkin quote, "Every Christian needs help and every Christian has some help to give"; Nate Larkin, *Samson and the Pirate Monks: Calling Men to Authentic Brotherhood* (United States: Thomas Nelson, 2007), 115.

When I say practice, I mean it. Making mistakes, building habits around it, everything that *practice* means. It takes a while. We've been invested in meeting our own needs in hiding, so coming out of hiding isn't easy. We have to build small skills to overcome the challenge, skills being consistent, coming to group, asking for help, and sharing our needs.

I run REV groups. There are also twelve-step groups, Pure Desire Groups, Celebrate Recovery groups, Samson groups, and more. Some have a fee, and some are free. Online groups have become more popular in the past few years, so there are lots of options. The goal is to find a group that's safe where you can be honest. You may need to visit more than one to find the right fit.

But there is nothing more important in early recovery than finding a good group. It helps you build the skills you need for long-term recovery faster.

CHAPTER 5

THE DARK NIGHT

I WAS STANDING AT THE DOORWAY OF MY home office, and I could see the cursor blinking in the search engine box. Six feet separated me from the computer. My heart was racing.

I had just connected to the internet for the first time in thirty days.

My wife was gone for the weekend in San Francisco. It was the first time that she was away since my secret had been exposed the month before.

It had been incredibly difficult over that month as I recounted the ways I had lied to her, the depth of my addiction, and even some of the content and sites that I visited.

She was totally hurt, understandably, and had a lot of questions. She was also loving and gracious to me. But it just took her being gone for a day or two before the old lure of the internet and pornography came back into focus.

I had tried to prepare myself for her being away. She took our computer modem with her to California. I met with a friend for dinner earlier, and I tried to watch a safe movie on my VCR. I tried to fill up my time, and I tried to structure it so there would be no room for temptation.

But I remembered an old modem in the basement that I had thought was once broken. *Could I get it working?* my obsessive mind thought. I spent an hour or more installing and playing with the drivers until I heard it connect.

The sound of the connection scared me. It was the same sound I had heard for hundreds of nights before. In the past, the very sound would excite me and make me feel alive. It signaled that the adventure of searching porn and masturbating were minutes away.

But the fear of what I was about to do made me jump up and stand at the door, one foot in the office and one foot in the hallway. *Am I going to do this?* I thought.

But a second thought came right after: *If I could destroy the modem, I'd be safe tonight.*

In the next moment, I ran to the kitchen and grabbed a hammer. Then I went back to the office.

I opened up the back of the tower computer, ripped out the newly installed modem, and began to smash it. The hard plastic didn't break easy. Minutes went by as I struggled to destroy it.

"Victory!" Or so I thought.

But I immediately sensed a dark presence in my apartment. I was gripped with fear like I was in a horror movie where you realize the killer is in the house.

I ran from room to room, turning on every light in the place. But no corner of the apartment felt safe. As I moved from one end of the building to the other, the darkness was everywhere.

I called my wife's cell phone in desperation. It was two o'clock in the morning for me, midnight for her. Luckily, she picked up the phone.

"What's wrong?" she asked.

I was filled with shame that I had even turned on the computer. I felt like I had already failed since I had agreed to not go online alone.

But in that moment, I was so scared. My words began to slur, and I started crying.

I told her the story. "I connected to the internet with an old modem . . ." I explained. "And now I am scared."

My wife, sensing something was wrong, immediately started praying for me. She prayed that I would feel safe. We talked for a few minutes, and she encouraged me. She thanked me for telling her and calling.

"If you're still scared after we hang up," she said. "Go stay at Jeff and Maggie's."

I hung up the phone, and for the next thirty seconds I felt okay. Then, all of a sudden, the presence was worse than ever. It was suffocating.

I grabbed some clothes and my bag and left within a minute.

It was three in the morning when I knocked on the door of my sister's apartment.

She didn't ask any questions and showed me to the couch, where I fell right to sleep.

The next day when I returned to the apartment with my brother-in-law, Jeff, all the lights were still on, but the presence was gone.

Nothing like this has ever happened to me before or since. What was the darkness? What was the evil presence? Was it my fear or some sort of panic attack?

I'm not sure. But when we go after the things that have trapped our heart, it is a fight. When we choose recovery, we upset the natural order of things in our life. "The natural life in each of us knows," C. S. Lewis writes, "that if the spiritual life gets hold of it, all its self-centeredness and self-will are going to be killed and it is ready to fight tooth and nail to avoid that."[1]

---

1. C. S. Lewis, *The Joyful* Christian (New York: Touchstone, 1996), 50.

Getting free means a power shift. The self-ish part of you that drives the porn behavior is no longer calling the shots. We experience pushback when we try to live a new way. Sometimes it's dramatic like my night in the apartment.

But more often it's subtle. The tempting voice within asks whether our favorite porn star has posted a new video on her Instagram.

For years, we have been invested in hanging on to and hiding porn. We've been entrenched in meeting our own needs. This has been our go to. This is our normal.

We have lost the power to choose. We blame the temptations and triggers in our life for our choices.

"My smart phone filter wasn't working"

"My accountability partner didn't call."

"The girl at the grocery store was showing cleavage."

"My hotel room had cable."

"I was horny, and my wife went to sleep early."

"But everyone is watching *Game of Thrones!*"

Add to a growing list of sites—such as Facebook, YouTube, Reddit, Twitter, and Instagram—engineered like slot machines to keep us online and clicking.

It's easy to blame these things.

But when we blame, we don't take ownership for our life. We misplace responsibility. The daily reality that it is paralyzing, life-threatening, and soul-crushing is lost on us.

After the night in my apartment, I knew I needed to take recovery seriously. The sheer power of the experience got my attention. Hitting rock bottom is a phrase used in recovery to describe a moment when you know you need help and can't do it alone. It's where you let go of all denial and start being honest with yourself. That night was my rock bottom.

Why are you reading this? Have you started to realize that porn has hijacked you? That it's your go-to escape? Stress release? Pain eraser?

Maybe you've had a scary encounter of your own.

I've heard of guys getting an anonymous letter through email that threatens legal action for something they've downloaded. Stories of guys being flagged by their IT department or, worse, fired for porn. I know of guys who were blackmailed by websites and cam girls.

Deep down we know there are offline consequences for our online behavior. But we willingly ignore the danger and continue.

"Most of us have two lives," Steven Pressfield writes. "The life we live and the unlived life within us. Between the two stands Resistance."[2]

Deep down, we know this is true.

We have been on the sidelines of our own life.

Are you closer to living the unlived life within, the one God intended for you? The one that taps into your full potential? Or is there still Resistance?

Steven Pressfield writes that "resistance is the most toxic force on the planet. It is the root of more unhappiness than poverty, disease, and erectile dysfunction. To yield to Resistance deforms our spirit. It stunts us and makes us less than we are and were born to be."[3]

That late night, I came face to face with my Resistance. It was obvious.

But most of the time it sneaks up on us in more subtle ways. It comes in the form of click-bait or in our obsessive thoughts. It hides in our procrastination and our isolation. It's in the feelings of entitlement or that double-look. Resistance does not go away. It's a dragon we must slay each day.

So how do we do this? Build up skills and tools to overcome Resistance? We need a plan. The days

2. Steven Pressfield, *The War of Art: Break Through the Blocks and Win Your Inner Creative Battles* (United States: Black Irish Entertainment LLC, 2002).
3. Pressfield, *The War of Art*.

of showing up and hoping we make the right decision in the moment are over.

We can't wait any longer for rock-bottom moments to prompt us in to action. They may come too late or never at all. We have to choose to take action.

CHAPTER 6

THE PORN FREE PLAN THAT NEVER FAILS

SO YOU MIGHT BE THINKING AT THIS POINT, How do I get this to work for me? I want to be porn free. What do I have to do?

I was on a writer's retreat recently, and I challenged myself to boil down recovery to the actual steps that guys have to take. I had read of an old self-help book by another Chicagoan, W. Clement Stone, called *The Success System That Never Fails.*[1] In it he makes a bold claim: if the system is followed it will lead to success and never to failure. I challenged myself to write a similar system for quitting porn.

---

1. W. Clement Stone, *The Success System That Never Fails* (Englewood Cliffs, N.J.: Prentice-Hall, 1962).

There are five steps that if practiced will lead to long-term freedom.

1. AWARENESS

At some point in our journey, we discover that porn is not working for us. Maybe we feel increasingly controlled by it. It's taking up more room in our life. It's dominating our thinking and free time. Or maybe we are getting bored with it. We find ourselves watching more and escalating to more extreme forms of porn to get the same level of excitement. The porn we looked at last year or a few years back doesn't do it for us now. Like the beer drinker who builds up a tolerance, we need something stronger to get the same buzz. A third possibility is porn is creating life consequences for us. It's impacting our relationships. We withdraw from our partner. When we do connect, we struggle to get and maintain an erection. It's putting our job at risk. We are more distracted and becoming increasingly paranoid that we are going to get caught. It isolates us. Our confidence and presence are diminished, and we feel alone.

No matter what the specifics are, there is a conflict growing within us. We know that porn is not working, but we keep going back to it. This is the essential awareness that is necessary to move forward.

We have an awareness that something is wrong. But we get stuck in two places: denial and the pursuit of self-knowledge.

You might be asking how can denial come after awareness? But there is a big difference between being aware of a problem and deciding to change.

I'm reminded of a concept I learned from coach Dan Sullivan: Imagine that you are standing on the edge of a dock, considering getting on a boat. You're straddling the boat and the dock with a foot on each.

But something keeps you on the dock. You think, *Is this really necessary?* Or maybe, *It's not that bad.*

"In some ways, they are in the worst of both worlds," coach Dan Sullivan writes. "A part of them wants to go on a boat ride, the other one wants to stay on the dock, and they refuse to make a decision."[2]

In denial, we procrastinate. We avoid making a decision about our awareness like putting off paying a bill that has come due. This delay comes from equal parts fear and pride.

The second way we get stuck is in the pursuit of self-knowledge. We watch videos, buy books, listen

---

2. Dan Sullivan, *The 4 C's Formula* (Toronto: The Strategic Coach Inc., 2015), 34.

to podcasts, and read posts on Reddit. We indulge the faint hope that we will discover how to use porn in a "safe way" without it controlling our life. We desperately want something that makes this okay.

When that option is exhausted, we search for a less painful way to quit. One that doesn't involve giving up things we like, looking bad, or asking for help.

Our assumption if we find the right article or idea, we'll do the right thing. We want to think ourselves into right action. But our relationship with porn comes with a habit that has been honed over years of repeated involvement. We have conditioned ourselves by returning to it, over and over.

Any useful knowledge we acquire is quickly overridden by our own desire and cravings. The AA Big Book says it best: "*Self-knowledge* availed us nothing." Our knowledge alone cannot change us.

Samuel Beckett wrote a play called *Waiting for Godot*. It's about two guys sitting around waiting for another guy. Spoiler alert: the other guy never shows up.

I could write a play called *Waiting for Recovery* about two guys sitting around talking about recovery, but not doing anything. Spoiler alert: recovery never comes.

Once we let go of the denial and the idea that we will be able to think our way out of this, we can move to step two.

2. CONNECTION

I grew up embracing the simple idea that "I take care of me." Many of us develop this habit of self-dependence growing up. Perhaps our parents were not there for us and a primary need went unmet. It could have been from a lack of consistency that made us doubt we would be cared for. We may have experienced separation or rejection early in life where we lose trust in depending on others.

This way of living based on my "I take care of me" mantra worked for me most of the time. It led to some early successes in school and life that reinforced my self-dependence. In fact, I thought of it as one of my strengths.

But it had one downside. When I encountered a circumstance in life that overwhelmed me, I would fall apart. I never wanted to ask for help.

This was particularly true with porn.

Porn and porn behaviors thrive in isolation. The secretive behavior actually fuels the excitement. And at its core, beneath the lust and orgasms, we are relying on ourselves to meet our own needs.

It fits perfectly with "I take care of me."

So even though we have a newfound awareness that this is not working for us—that we need to let go of porn—the idea of bringing others into our private world is terrifying.

I had a coaching client once say his goal was not perfection. He said, "I just don't want to look bad."

This is our predicament; we want to do what it takes and quit porn. But we also don't want to look bad.

This sets up in us a competing commitment. You cannot be committed to both. Whichever you associate with more pain and cost, you *will* do.

For many of us, the fear of looking bad trumps doing what it takes.

The first recovery group I ever attended was called Redeemed Lives and was led by a warm and lively Anglican priest named Mario.

In the first few minutes of his talk, he quoted G. K. Chesterton. "Anything worth doing," he said, "is worth doing badly."[3]

Something about this phrase excited me. In my attempts prior to this group to quit porn, I had tried everything but looking bad. I avoided telling people about my problem. I hid it from my wife. I tried to figure it out in secret. And I failed over and over.

As Mario told stories of his own addictions and broken relationships with vulnerability and empathy, I immediately felt safe.

It reminds me of a quote I heard from one of my podcast guests Angus Nelson. "Whenever you show

---

3. Adapted from the original G. K. Chesterton quote, *What's Wrong with the World*, 320.

yourself vulnerable," he said. "You give others permission to do the same."

I had permission from Mario's honest confession to be vulnerable. I could stop pretending I had it all together and minimizing how much I was hiding and hurting.

I wanted God to zap me so I would stand up to temptation and stop wanting to look at porn. Instead, I sat in front of Mario, with his black suit and white collar, realizing that this was what I needed.

"The opposite of addiction is not sobriety," Johann Hari remarked in his 2015 TED talk. "The opposite of addiction is connection."[4]

For me it was not humiliating or shameful to be at the group, like I feared. It was more like breathing after being trapped below the surface of water. Or discovering a freshwater source on a dry summer hike. I didn't realize how thirsty I was until I started to drink.

I had been so painfully alone in my struggle. I didn't even know what it meant to be in community as I sat in my small group that night and made a painful account of my journey to this point with pornography. I showed up. I was vulnerable. The

---

4. Johann Hari, "Everything You Think You Know about Addiction Is Wrong," TED Talks, June 2015, https://www.ted.com/talks/johann _hari_everything_you_think_you_know_about_addiction_is_ wrong#t-202527.

transformation in me was beginning. I was fully on board the boat and had left the shore. I decided to change.

Even now as you start to think about what it would take to be porn free, you can easily start to get overwhelmed with the how.

Dan Sullivan and Benjamin Hardy speak to this concept directly in their book *Who Not How*.

Instead of asking "How can I accomplish this?" they write, "A much better question is: 'Who can help me achieve this?'"[5]

You may not know right now who can help you. And that's okay. But I want you to start to think about this now. Other people help us move from self-dependence and denial, into real recovery. They also expand the tools and resources that are available to us. They witness and help take ownership for our goals and commitments.

Once we have honest connection, we can then move to step three.

3. A PLAN

When guys contact me they typically have a goal of going porn free. Sometimes they have a

5. Benjamin Hardy, Dan Sullivan, *Who Not How: The Formula to Achieve Bigger Goals Through Accelerating Teamwork* (United States: Hay House, 2020), 7–8.

sobriety date in mind. Six months or a year or forever . . . which is a huge goal.

I love what James Clear said in his book *Atomic Habits*.

Clear shares his approach to achieving the things we want in life. "Forget about goals," he writes. "Focus on systems instead."[6]

It's a simple idea.

Goals are based on the result we want. For example, being porn free for one year.

But systems are the processes that create the result we want—i.e., our recovery plan, our active commitments, our accountability group, etc.

"If you're having trouble changing your habits, the problem isn't you," he writes. "The problem is your system."[7]

This is hopeful news if you have been struggling. Your goal isn't the problem. You *can* do this. But getting the right systems in place is the key.

Now when I ask new guys in coaching about their plan, they typically share about a tool they have tried.

---

6. James Clear, *Atomic Habits: Tiny Changes, Remarkable Results: an Easy & Proven Way to Build Good Habits & Break Bad Ones* (United States: Penguin Random House, 2018), 23.

7. James Clear, *Atomic Habits*, 27.

Examples:

- I installed a filter.
- I don't keep my smartphone on the bedside table.
- I meet with an accountability partner.
- I have a morning routine.
- I take cold showers.

It's an action they have taken. But it's not a system.

The recovery plan I recommend is a system. It's made up of specific commitments and statements that define your recovery.

I have coached millionaires, high-ranking military officers, executives, doctors, and pastors. In their normal life, they build businesses, reach BIG goals, and lead others. They can plan. They can implement.

But when it comes to their internal recovery work, they experience repeated failure. They make the same mistakes over and over and expect different results.

For much of my life I believed the lie that I did not have "self-discipline." Like it was the sole domain of Navy Seals and internet billionaires.

But in recovery I realized that discipline came from my habits.

"The trick is," Gary Keller writes, "choose the right habit and bring just enough discipline to establish it."[8]

The more the habit becomes part of your life, the easier it is to maintain. And the more people see you being consistent with a habit, the more disciplined you appear.

SO HOW DO YOU BUILD A RECOVERY PLAN? YOU BUILD A NEW SYSTEM.

You look at the areas of your life where you need to grow and find the right habits to support that growth.

Everything in your plan has to have a why, a reason for doing it. And committing to the right habits is crucial.

I once coached an ultra-marathon runner. He was super disciplined.

We identified a big need for him: connection. He was really isolated and did not have any guys in his life supporting him.

---

8. Gary Keller, Jay Papasan, *The One Thing: The Surprisingly Simple Truth Behind Extraordinary Results* (United States: Bard Press, 2013).

When I asked about what he did for self-care in his life, guess what his answer was? He ran.

I asked, "Do you ever run with people?"

He said no because of his running pace and training plan. At the time he was running over ten hours a week alone. So his biggest self-care investment did not meet one of his biggest needs.

That system was doomed to fail.

I have created a video for you to create a thirty-day plan at https://pornfreebook.com/resources.

Watch it now or when you finish reading the book.

BRIEFLY, HERE'S WHAT I RECOMMEND FOR A 30-DAY PLAN

YOUR WHY

First and foremost, you need clarity about why you are doing this. You need to tap into your internal reason for going porn free. And it may not be what you think. Common answers guys give for going porn free include my wife, my marriage, my faith in God, my family, etc. These are good reasons, but they are external. For your why, we need to go deeper. See the appendix at the end of this book to develop your "Why" statement.

EMOTIONAL TRIGGERS, MISTAKEN BELIEFS, AND WEAK LINKS

If we see addiction as an "extreme version of a habit,"[9] recovery is the process of transforming our habits.

In order to change, we have to focus on the areas where we need to grow. These come down to three things:

1. Emotional Triggers
2. Mistaken Beliefs
3. Weak Links

Let me share a quick illustration.

I always hated being alone. I remember coming home from work as a single guy on Friday nights. The front door would close, and I would think to myself, "Now what?" When I was alone, an emptiness would come over me. It didn't matter how many friends I had or activities I was involved in. Being alone always triggered me. When I was alone, I would hear this lie on repeat: "Nobody can see you, so nobody loves you." I hated the feeling it produced. All I wanted was to escape it. So 95 percent

---

9. Horvath, *Sex, Drugs, Gambling, and Chocolate*, 1.

of the time—and that's probably understating it—this feeling would lead me to acting out with porn on my computer.

What was happening? I was responding to an emotional trigger—the feeling of being alone. This led to me subconsciously agreeing with this belief: "Nobody can see you, so nobody loves you." So the emotional trigger tapped into a mistaken belief that was already there.

Finally, I had a weak link: my computer. It was unprotected back then. I didn't have any filter software on it. I didn't have accountability or boundaries, so it was easy to slip into a binge whenever I engaged craving.

Notice that pattern: there was an emotional trigger, there was a mistaken belief, and there was a weak link. I can't tell you how many nights that pattern defined my life.

You know another word for patterns that define your life? Habits.

Through years of porn use, I had created powerful habits around my certain feelings and thoughts. When I experienced an emotional trigger, it would lead to agreeing with mistaken beliefs and conclusions. At this point, I would engage craving.

A favorite quote of mine comes from the Freedom Model for Addictions. "Craving is NOT something that happens to you; it's something you actively do."[10]

A simple way of looking at craving is thinking that porn or a porn behavior would feel good right now. My craving did not come from external sources like women and sexy TV shows. It was a habit that came from within.

Growing up, there was a popular beer commercial for Miller beer. It showed guys working hard during the day and then finishing up. Then the guys punched out on the time clock, cleaned up, put their tools away, and flipped the closed sign on the shop. It was *Miller Time*. It was that time of the day to head to the bar, grab a cold one, and reward yourself with a beer.

This is the habit for us. We encounter an emotional trigger. It could even come from the end of the hard day's work like the commercial. And at some level, we start heading toward our own version of *Miller Time*—only for us, it's with porn and porn behaviors.

Finally, our Weak Links are the things in our environment that make it easy to use porn.

Whether it's our bedtime habits, our phones, our computers, our smart TVs, our streaming subscriptions, our social media—if porn is always a

---

10. Mark Scheeren, Michelle Dunbar, Steven Slate, *The Freedom Model for Addictions: Escape the Treatment and Recovery Trap* (Netherlands: BRI Publishing, 2017), 59.

click away for us, it's hard to change our habits. Especially with powerful emotional triggers. We're like the recently recovered alcoholic who still has a fridge stocked with beer.

Examples of Emotional Triggers:

- Being alone
- Boredom
- Depression
- Exhaustion
- Anxiety or stress
- Entitlement
- Resentment or anger
- Rejection
- Needing physical touch
- Desiring intimacy
- Longing for nurture
- Wanting to be seen

Examples of Mistaken Beliefs:

- There's something wrong with me.
- I'm unseen or forgotten.
- I'm unlovable.
- I can't change. I can never change.
- I'm not good enough.
- I'm a failure.
- Nobody likes me. Nobody could like me.
- If people knew the real me, they'd reject me.

- I hate myself. I deserve to hate myself.
- I'm hopeless.
- I've never been good with discipline.
- I'm worthless.
- I'm a loser.
- I deserve a break.
- A little bit won't hurt me.
- If I can't do this perfectly, then I can't do it at all.
- My stupid brain is addicted to porn.
- I'm ugly. I'm unattractive. Nobody could want me.
- Don't all guys look at porn?

Examples of Weak Links:

- No filtered internet
- Too many connected devices
- A smartphone always within three feet
- Social media sites
- Late night TV/gaming/streaming
- YouTube
- The feeling of unaccountable time
- Traveling without a plan

So your plan needs to identify Emotional Triggers, Mistaken Beliefs, and Weak Links.

- What feelings or emotions most often trigger you?

- What are the most common thoughts or beliefs that go through your head that lead to craving?
- What in your environment makes it easy to use porn?

ACTIVE COMMITMENTS

Once you identify some of these challenges, you create commitments in your plan mapped to these growth areas.

"To break a habit," coach Craig Perra says, "you have to make a habit."[11]

The key is your new habits need to be mapped to your biggest challenges. This plan is not just a "go to the gym and eat healthier" plan. It's an active commitment to improve the areas that directly contribute to your porn habit.

If you identify loneliness as an emotional trigger, it might be a habit supported by joining a group. If it's fighting with a spouse, it may be committing to marriage counseling or taking a marriage class. If it's managing work stress, it may be creating a new routine for planning your work day.

---

11. Craig Perra, "Craig's Story," The Mindful Habit, https://www
.themindfulhabit.com/about-craig-perra/.

I recommend starting with no more than three new habits for a new plan. Focus on creating consistency over intensity. A small habit that you stick to over thirty days will yield better results than a big commitment you give up in week one.

If done right, your plan will start to look like the personal development plan for a growth-minded, healthy person. It will reflect more of who you are becoming in your life, not just the behaviors you are avoiding.

One final tool I encourage is creating a consequence and reward for your plan.

A consequence is a pre-commitment you make in your plan that you will implement if you use porn. A reward is used as an incentive to mark a successful thirty days of building new habits, following through with commitments, and staying porn free.

You can find more on consequence and reward including examples online at https://pornfreebook .com/resources.

Once you have a draft of a plan, it's time to move to step four.

4. ACTIVATION

Your plan is activated when you share it with someone. That's when it gets real.

I have actually seen guys stay stuck at step three for months. Polishing and refining their plan. Tweaking it. But never sharing it and never starting. A plan that has not been committed to in some cases is worse than no plan at all. It's a form of advanced denial where you are still trying to do this alone or avoid looking bad.

Activating your plan with someone else is a decision. It's when you jump into the boat and leave the comfort of shore.

Mental toughness coach, Chris Dorris, speaks of it this way: "The decision had been made and all that was left to do was whatever it took," he says. "And that involved no consideration. There was no more deliberation."[12]

By sharing your plan, you move from the deliberation phase of recovery to the ALL-IN phase. No more hiding. No more procrastination. You are now *committed*.

You might be thinking, "Does it have to be activated by sharing it? Can't someone just choose to follow a plan?"

Yes and no. I am sure there are some people who one day wake up and decide they are done looking at porn.

---

12. Christopher Dorris, *All IN!*, audio course (United States: The Dorris Group, 2011).

I had a friend who was like this who read about sex-trafficking and the online porn industry. He was so moved by it and so deeply connected with the raw truth of the article that he decided to never look at porn again.

And it worked.

But that's not you. Think back to the habits you have created and the relationship you have formed with porn over your lifetime. These do not go away overnight. Old habits indeed die hard.

You can totally find freedom. I believe one hundred percent in that statement. But if you could have just decided to quit it would have happened by now.

So, you need to build some new skills to overcome this challenge. One of the most powerful habits you can create is the practice of making commitments in front of another human being. Some people call this accountability. I call it ownership.

Your plan outlines your commitment to be porn free. It defines your personal why statement. It prioritizes your growth areas and the habits you are building to support growth. It spells out your specific commitments including consequences and rewards for the period of the plan.

If you do share it with an "accountability partner" or your spouse, they actually know what you are actively committed to doing to stay porn free rather than just a passive commitment to *not* do a behavior.

Remember this about your system. Porn free days are a by-product of your system.

So what makes this plan never fail? How can I even make such a bold claim?

For that we must go to the fifth and final step.

5. REVIEW

In the military after any mission, they have an after-action review (AAR). An AAR is a debrief process where we analyze what happened, and how it can be done better. More specifically how it can be done better by the people who are responsible for it.

So who's responsible for your plan? You are.

Depending on who you are working with, this review can be monthly, weekly, or even daily. You take ownership for talking about how it went.

YOUR F.A.S.T. AFTER-ACTION REVIEW
(ADAPTED FROM MILTON S. MAGNESS)

F - What powerful *feelings* and emotions came up for me?

A - How did I do with my **active commitments** and habits? Did they happen? Why or why not?

S - Were there any **slips** in my plan? Did I engage any craving or mistaken beliefs? Did I do any unsound activities? Did I skip an important commitment or habit?

T - What new or upcoming **threats** am I aware of? (Magness refers to threats as "situations that require tools.")[13]

The last point of the After-Action Review hints at the power of review. We are creating a system that develops awareness. What's working, what's not, what needs to be improved, what's next? If you identify a threat, what tool are you going to use to deal with it? The only way this plan fails is if you skip the fifth step of review. Because no improvement comes without new awareness.

---

13. Milton S. Magness, *Stop Sex Addiction: Real Hope, True Freedom for Sex Addicts and Partners* (United States: Central Recovery Press, 2013).

After review, our newfound awareness takes us back to the first step of our plan.

Awareness leads us to form **Connection**. There we improve our **Plan** and **Activate** it. Our next **Review** generates new awareness. The process repeats.

Samuel Beckett penned this quote in his play *Westward Ho.*

"Ever tried. Ever failed. No matter. Try Again. Fail again. Fail better."[14]

The way we improve is not to never fail again. It's to fail better. It's in the commitment to continual improvement that freedom comes.

I don't know your challenges or how long your road to freedom will take. But I do know this plan, if you choose to follow it, will always lead to success and never to failure.

---

14. Samuel Beckett, *Worstward Ho* (United Kingdom: John Calder, 1983).

CHAPTER 7

THE ENEMY OF RECOVERY IS SELF-REJECTION

FINDING TRUE FREEDOM IS NOT JUST QUIT-ting a bad habit, it's about discovering the real you. My biggest breakthrough came after an epic failure.

One memory that stands out was when I was unemployed for a few months, and I was doing a job search. When you're unemployed, there's kind of this loneliness and a lot of rejection. You have to continue to affirm your worth, that you are a good employee, that you have good skills. Because you're home alone, you are susceptible to that lie that you're worthless or that you're not hirable. I was really feeling that.

I had tried to keep myself safe. I had a plan. I was not using my computer at home. I didn't have Internet access at home. I was going to my parents' house at the time and was doing job searches. I'd go and search and send emails and all that type of stuff during the day, and then I'd come back to my house in the evening.

It was still the first couple years of my recovery, and the feelings of loneliness and rejection were becoming unmanageable for me. I figured out a way to act out. I downloaded a short video and burned it to a VCD. A VCD was a CD-ROM that could play in a DVD player. I took it home and watched it.

I immediately felt ashamed. I knew I had to tell my wife. I sat her down and said I had something to tell her. Right then she knew where we were going with this conversation, and she started to cry. I explained what had happened. I didn't make excuses about unemployment or rejection. I just told her the facts.

She was upset and there was a lot of hurt in her face. I could see the actual consequences of my choices and how they affected her. It was heartbreaking.

She started to ask some questions, and something welled up in me from a deep place in my gut. I turned away from her. I was so ashamed I began to bend into myself, hiding my face in the couch. I started to weep. Through the tears a question came to me, and I repeated it over and over: "Why? Why? Why?"

This was so dramatic that my wife was surprised. She saw me in pain and said, "What are you asking?"

Between the sobs, I finally got it out. "Why do you love me?"

At my core, I became aware that I felt unlovable. I felt damaged and disqualified. Not good enough. That feeling came before my relationship with pornography. It went deeper and further back. In fact, pornography was my escape from this feeling. It was my way of numbing this core lie that I had believed about myself—that I was unlovable.

My wife just started affirming me. She told me the ways she loved me, and she prayed for me.

A significant event marked me growing up. Right before my third birthday, my mom gave birth to my brother John. But John was born with heart complications and died a few days after his birth. I have no memories of his death or the time when he was alive. But in the two years after his death, my family suffered. My mom was sad, and my dad threw himself into his ministry.

Kids are generally bad interpreters of what is going on around them. I internalized two things from my brother's death: my mom's sadness and my dad's absence. I made them about me.

I started hiding my needs and trying to manage on my own. But here was the problem: deep down, I craved people's affirmation and love.

I began to agree with the mistaken belief that I could only depend on myself. This set me up. I experienced a lot of pain and confusion in those early years. Displaced grief. Fierce self-reliance. The older I got, the more this feeling of being unlovable defined my experience.

When I discovered pornography, it provided an escape and that numbing to that feeling of being unlovable. A few years back, I read *Tattoos on the Heart: The Power of Boundless Compassion* by Father Gregory Boyle.

Father Boyle works in Los Angeles with ex-gang members in a restorative process to take people out of gangs and help them recover their lives. "The self cannot survive without love," he quotes James Gilligan. "And the self, starved of love, dies."[1]

This is a powerful idea. How does this tie into compulsive porn use, though?

Underneath the lust and hunger, we are looking for affirmation. We're looking for love. Pornography's lure is that it offers a substitute for the intimacy we desire.

---

1. Gregory Boyle, *Tattoos on the Heart* (New York: Free Press, 2010), 46.

After another relapse in my recovery, I went to a counseling intensive with a therapist in Colorado. His name was Mike Pinkston. Mike gave me an exercise to journal about. He asked me to write about a particular type of porn I liked and then journal about the needs I was looking to meet in that expression of porn.

When I was back at the hotel, I started thinking. The first type of pornography that came to mind involved a distinct ethnic group. The women in this genre were slightly older than me as well.

It surprised me a bit. I did not have a go-to type of porn, but this example would work for the exercise. I asked myself, "What need was I looking to fill?"

A simple idea jumped into my head. Nurture.

This particular ethnic group has a soothing way of speaking. There is a softness and calm to the tones that reminded me of the way a mother would speak to a newborn. As I journaled more, I wrote that I wanted to be cared for and seen. I wanted nurture and love.

Could it be any clearer?

I had eroticized a real need and projected it onto the pictures of these women.

I began to think of other turn-ons. One by one, I uncovered the needs underneath.

I thought of how I was drawn to voluptuous women whose bodies seemed designed to provide nurture and warmth. To have a woman like this would make me feel enough.

I thought of a porn star with sparkling eyes whose gaze would always make me feel seen.

Even the ridiculous premises of pornography played into my desires. They invited me into a fantasy of feminine intimacy, where I was the object of adoration. Where I was wanted. This pull can still be powerful in my life.

I make it a rule to go to bed with my wife each night. This habit was born out the experience of early recovery where unaccountable time at night was a real threat to my sobriety. I have kept this habit for many years. It's still wise, and it helps me get more sleep.

One night recently, she went to bed early and without me. I started channel surfing.

I stopped the clicker on a reality show with famous celebrity women. They were shopping for clothes. I was sucked in particularly by one of the women. I know very little about her, but she is pretty and very feminine. I watched transfixed and in a haze.

Then it occurred to me: what need am I trying to meet here? My wife had gone to bed early so I felt lonely but also rejected. It was subtle, but it was there.

"It's nearly inevitable," Gay Hendricks writes. "That you will someday encounter a boulder in the living room of your Zone of Genius. That boulder is the belief that you are unlovable. This false belief fuels the frantic search for something external to yourself that confirms you are indeed lovable."[2]

In that moment, watching the reality show, I realized I was agreeing with the lie that I was unlovable. And I was lying to myself that this woman and the image of her body would somehow make me feel better.

I turned off the TV, not because of rules or sheer will power, but because I am unwilling to agree with the lie.

OUR GREATEST TRAP IN LIFE

Henri Nouwen, another Catholic priest, authored one of my favorite books, *Life of the Beloved*. It's a series of letters to a friend named Fred Bratman, who was a reporter and journalist. Fred was a secular guy who wrote for *The New Yorker* and sparked up a friendship with Nouwen.

At some point, Fred said to Nouwen, "Hey, could you write a book for someone like me who lives in a secular world and isn't a person of faith? Can you write something that will help me?"

2. Gay Hendricks, *The Big Leap: Conquer Your Hidden Fear and Take Life to the Next Level* (United Kingdom: HarperCollins, 2009), 155.

What does Nouwen write Fred? He boils it down to one idea: you are beloved.

"All I want to say to you is this," Nouwen writes. "You are the beloved and all I can hope that you can hear these words as spoken to you with all the tenderness of force that love can hold. My only desire is to make these words reverberate in every corner of your being. You are the beloved."[3]

He gets this word *beloved* specifically from a story in the Bible where Jesus is being baptized by John the Baptist. It says a voice from heaven came and said, "You are my son, the beloved, my favor rests on you" (Luke 3:22). God himself speaks of his love of his son, Jesus, and he calls him the beloved.

What Nouwen argues is that we're all beloved. That is the core of our existence. We were created by our Creator and he loves us with the same love that he spoke about Jesus. "You are my son, the beloved, my favor rests on you"—that is for all of us. It is in our DNA that we are beloved. It's the core of our identity.

Admittedly, there is a theological perspective there that you have to buy into. But just hear this thing, this idea that at our core we are lovable. Our identity is not based on what we've done, but on the

3. Henri Nouwen, *Life of the Beloved* (New York: Crossroad Publishing Company, 1992).

fact that we are beloved by our Creator. We are lovable because we bear the imprint of our Creator.

Nouwen goes on to say that our greatest trap in life is not addiction. It's not focusing on greed or other sorts of prideful activities. It's self-rejection.

He writes:

"As soon as someone accuses me or criticizes me, as soon as I am rejected, left alone, or abandoned, I find myself thinking, 'Well, that proves once again that I am a nobody.'... [My dark side says,] I am no good...I deserve to be pushed aside, forgotten, rejected, and abandoned. Self-rejection is the greatest enemy of the spiritual life because it contradicts the sacred voice that calls us the 'Beloved.' Being the Beloved constitutes the core truth of our existence."[4]

This lines up with my experience. Every time I sought porn to cover that lie that I was unlovable, it actually left me feeling more abandoned and more rejected. That statement, "Well, that proves once again that I'm a nobody" is what I felt like after every time I acted out.

When my wife caught me looking at porn all those years ago, and as I started telling people about my addiction and my struggles, a strange thing

---

4. Henri Nouwen, *Life of the Beloved* (New York: Crossroad Publishing Company, 1992).

happened. People heard what I said, heard what I shared, and started expressing their love for me. With my hiding out of the way, I was able to receive more of their love. I even started feeling more of God's love.

Many times, I remember sitting in church in the back row feeling like a second-class Christian because no matter how much I sang about God's love for me in worship, I felt unlovable. At my core, I had fallen into the greatest trap in life. Why *would* anyone love me? Why *would* God love me? Why *would* my friends love me? Why *would* my wife love me?

Porn perpetuated this lie. And I continue to reject myself when I agree with it.

Right now, I just want you to take in that word *beloved*. Take that whole verse in: "You are my son, the beloved, my favor rests on you." There's a still, small voice that says, "You are beloved." It's part of your DNA. It's part of your core existence.

My only desire is to make these words reverberate in every corner of your being: you are the beloved. That no matter what you've done with porn or your broken attempts to find love, you are still lovable.

"It's obviously that our brokenness is often," Nouwen writes, "most painfully experienced with respect to our sexuality. . . . Our sexuality reveals to us our enormous yearning for communion, the desires of our body to be touched, embraced, and safely held belong to the deepest longings of our heart."[5]

5. Nouwen, *Life of the Beloved*.

CHAPTER 8
SELF-CARE

I ASKED MY REV GROUP THIS QUESTION: "What is self-care?"

I assumed their answers would be physical—working out, getting the right amount of sleep, or something about habits. But one by one as they shared, a theme emerged about compassion. Being kind to yourself. Recognizing your worth. Investing in restorative activities.

It rang true. The days early in recovery were hard. I was living in a new way, and I was feeling my feelings. I remember being at Starbucks one morning after a relapse. I was still feeling ashamed of the night before.

"How are you?" asked Kevin, my favorite barista.

"Fine," I said.

Only, the question stuck with me. *How am I?* I'm not fine. I'm not fine at all. I'm a mess.

I exited the store quickly as tears came to my eyes. I felt ashamed from the night before, but I also felt broken.

Relapses are particularly confusing especially when you have had some distance from porn. We are flooded with feelings of failure. We are tempted to agree that we are hopeless.

Well, that didn't work, we think to ourselves. *I guess this is who I am.*

But the truth is this is a delicate process, and we need grace.

For years, we have lived in black-and-white thinking regarding porn. We go back and forth between two extremes: being consumed with porn and lust, or filled with shame and regret. Neither state is freedom.

Many guys from a faith background internalize that God is angry with them for their repeated failures. I remember avoiding church after a slip with pornography, thinking that I could go back only if I could get seven days clean.

In the fourteenth century, there was a group of zealous Christians called the Flagellants who would whip themselves in bizarre public rituals. They believed this act of self-punishment would make them right with God. This is an extreme comparison, but we do the same thing.

We judge ourselves. We self-punish. We agree with shame. We curse ourselves. I once was working with a pastor who had a relapse. His sense of shame was magnified by his position and calling. "This is unacceptable," he said. "I am a disgrace." He went on demeaning himself. The harshness of his words was sharp and jagged. He had nothing kind to say.

I then asked him to tell me what he would say in pastoral counseling if a man said these things about himself.

He was filled with compassion at the thought, but he could not transfer it to his own situation. When we think of others, we have grace, but our internal perfectionism and self-reliance cannot accept it for ourselves.

Learning self-care is a skill that can be built, but it is not modeled well by other men. Very few men are adept at knowing their needs and taking care of them.

> "When you seem to lose all you thought you had gained, do not despair. . . . You must expect setbacks and regressions. Don't say to yourself "All is lost. I have to start all over again." This is not true. What you have gained you have gained. . . . When you return to the

road, you return to the place where you left it, not to where you started."

—Henri Nouwen[1]

I am always saying things like, "You need self-care after a relapse," or "What kind of self-care do you have in your plan?" I even refer to porn as "unhealthy self-care." But what exactly is self-care and why do we need it?

I'll answer that question, but first I want to tell you about my favorite chair.

A few years back, my wife and I were driving back home from a family barbecue.

"Hey, can we stop at the furniture outlet?" my wife asked. "I'm looking for a chair that matches our living room."

We were on a tight budget at the time. We hadn't planned for a new piece of furniture. This outlet was cheap, but so was the furniture quality.

"There's a Salvation Army near there," I suggested. "Why don't we stop by and see if there's something we can use temporarily."

At the Salvation Army, we found an armchair. It was comfortable and it looked brand new. It even matched our color scheme.

It was marked fifty dollars.

"What do you think?" I asked.

---

1. Henri J. M. Nouwen, *The Inner Voice of Love: A Journey Through Anguish to Freedom* (New York: Doubleday, 1998), 38.

"I like it. It's a steal."

It gets better. It was Saturday, half-priced furniture day at the Salvation Army. The chair came to twenty-five dollars plus tax.

As I'm loading the chair into our minivan, I look at the brand under the cushion and Google it. This chair sells for about a thousand dollars new. And it was in great condition; it looked like it had never been used. We ended up with a thousand-dollar chair that cost twenty-five bucks.

This chair has become my favorite chair to read in, to pray in, to write. It sits in the living room by the fireplace. There is no TV in the room, so it's a place to think without distraction. I have recorded podcasts in it. When company comes over, I like to sit in it to talk to people. I led a Bible study from it. I have even taken naps in the chair.

To me, this chair symbolizes a place in my house where I get good self-care. Where I do things that are reflective, where I do things that are relational, where I do things that are restorative, and where I do things that are growth oriented.

Do you have a place like this in your life?

Let's start with a simple idea of what self-care is. Self-care is the process of identifying needs and taking the steps to meet them.

At the beginning, it's hard to see our real needs. They are obscured by the shame of our porn use.

What's more, the habit of going to porn is a quick reflex and it feels automatic.

But I have a simple tool for figuring out what our needs are. It's called the Feeling Wheel, first developed by author Gloria Willcox.[2] I created a modified version tailored for recovery. (Download it at https://pornfreebook.com/resources.)

The Feeling Wheel has six core feelings: Sad, Mad, Scared, Joyful, Powerful, and Peaceful. Underneath are descriptive words that help identify what we are feeling.

For example, feeling bored is a common one. It's under Sad because it points to a lack of excitement and happiness with current circumstances.

Rejected is under Scared. When we feel rejected, we're uncertain where we stand. Discontentment and fear are stirred up in us. We don't feel good enough.

Entitled is a feeling that often gives a green light to acting out with porn. It's under Mad, because it usually comes from the frustration of not getting something we think we deserve.

What's the connection between feelings and needs?

---

2. Gloria Willcox, "The Feeling Wheel: A Tool for Expanding Awareness of Emotions and Increasing Spontaneity and Intimacy," *Sage Journals* 12, no. 4 (October 1, 1982), 274-76, https://doi.org/10.1177/036215378201200411.

All feelings point to needs. Feelings are neither good nor bad. We have a tendency to focus a lot on what we consider "negative" feelings, especially when trying to improve ourselves. But there are plenty of examples where being sad, mad, or scared is the right thing to do.

Whenever the discussion of needs comes up, I think of Maslow's hierarchy of needs, named for Abraham Maslow, an American psychologist. Most of his writing and research was on what motivated humans. His theory of motivation is presented in his book *Motivation and Personality*.[3] Maslow was primarily interested in what makes people achieve their potential.

He was drawn to study people like Franklin Delano Roosevelt, Einstein, and impressionist painters like Renoir. Lincoln, Jefferson, and George Washington Carver were also subjects of his interest.

He developed the idea that humans were motivated by their needs. In order to achieve a high level of performance and mastery, they had to meet a number of needs first.

That's where the hierarchy comes in. It's commonly drawn as a pyramid. We move from base-level, simple needs to more complex, existential needs the higher we go.

---

3. Abraham H. Maslow, *Motivation and Personality* (New York: Harper & Row, 1981).

While Maslow's understanding of needs has influenced psychology for several generations, I have included one wild card in this mix. It's an additional need that comes from author and speaker Tony Robbins. It's particularly relevant when considering our ongoing fascination with using porn.

PHYSIOLOGICAL

Breathing, food, water, sleep, excretion, etc., make up the base of the pyramid. These are basic bodily functions we need to survive.

SAFETY

The second level is safety. It's our security, our sense of being. It can be tied to our employment, our resources, our physical home, our family structure. It's our health. It's the basics of what makes us feel secure.

VARIETY / UNCERTAINTY

This is the Tony Robbins addition to Maslow's list of needs.[4] Variety, or uncertainty, is the spice of life.

---

4. Anthony Robbins, "The Six Human Needs," *Anthony Robbins' Personal Power II: The Driving Force!* (San Diego: Robbins Research International Inc., 1996), Compact Disc no. 23.

Once we are confident of our safety and security, we start looking for adventure. Experiences like roller coasters, travel, trying new foods, and even horror movies create surprise and spark joy in our life.

LOVE AND BELONGING

That's our friendships, our romances, and our family. It can be the tribe that we're a part of, who we identify with, who we connect with. It also encompasses sexual intimacy.

ESTEEM

The next level up is esteem. Self-esteem, confidence, and achievement are all part of this level. It's the respect we feel from others, it's how we're seen, how we're perceived, but also where we feel appreciated and our work is valued.

SELF-ACTUALIZATION

This top level is the one Maslow was most interested in. That's when we have resolved our deficient needs like food and safety. We have built healthy connection with others, in our tribe, or in relationships. We our comfortable in our own skin. And we turn our focus to growth. This is where we start achieving our potential in our thinking and actions. It's where creativity, productivity, and mastery come from.

Maslow admitted that people aren't perfect. Some of these high performers that he was looking at could have problems in lower areas.

However, overall, they had resolved a lot of those smaller and simpler needs in order to achieve their great results.

He also said that despite the hierarchy, it was possible to feel some higher levels without lower ones. For example, you might feel a lack of security because you lose a job, but you have a great family and support system around you, so you still feel love and belonging.

Likewise, you could be secure financially, but going through a messy divorce where you don't feel the sense of belonging. You would feel a lot of disconnection and isolation.

You might have esteem in your life, but you might not feel loved at a certain level.

We can get to higher levels of need, but sometimes crises in our life can make a lower-level need become more important.

Let's break down a couple of these needs in terms of recovery.

We'll begin with physiological.

PHYSIOLOGICAL

You've probably heard that when you are feeling tempted, you should ask yourself, "Am I feeling hungry, angry, lonely, or tired?" H.A.L.T. for short. That hardly covers everything you could be feeling. I once joked it could stand for Horny, Anxious, Lazy, or Tense. The point is we need to first look at lower-level physiological need that isn't being met. In the case of hunger or in the case of tiredness, we might have a deprivation that we need to address.

For instance, consider when we are sleep deprived. Pornography struggles thrive late at night when we need rest. We need to go to bed and sleep. Instead, we're attempting to get rest through porn. Then we end up staying up later, which creates more fatigue. It has the opposite effect.

When I say that porn is unhealthy self-care, I mean that it often doesn't fulfill the need we try to meet with it. If we really need to go to sleep but we're staying up late clicking on links and looking at videos, it feels like self-care, but the need remains unmet.

SAFETY

Why do you have locks on your door at home, have anti-lock brakes in your car, or wear a helmet when you're on your bike? It's about safety. Similar to creating a safe home, we need to take responsibility for creating safety in our environment for recovery.

A big shift for me was when I started seeing my recovery choices as creating safety in my life rather than losing freedom or restricting me.

There's a part of us that needs and longs for safety, especially if we've been vulnerable in an area.

I remember once having my wife add a passcode to our basement TV. She restricted all R-rated and MA programming on our cable. The moment she set the code, I felt relief, not deprivation.

When we're constantly living in an environment that's unsafe, it creates anxiety in us. And that anxiety can even be an emotional trigger for us.

Do everything you can to create safety in your home and in other areas you can control in your world. The safety will lead to a calmer mind.

VARIETY / UNCERTAINTY

One of my favorite Bing Crosby lines comes from *White Christmas*: "Surely you know everybody's got a little bit of larceny in them."

At some point we all want to play the rebel. Blaise Pascal says we have an instinct that compels us to seek amusement and excitement. It's an escape from boredom and the reminders of our unhappiness. We are drawn to adventure and distraction. And often, "we like the chase," Pascal writes. "Better than the quarry."[5]

Porn so clearly fits this need. It offers endless variety and novelty. The escape fantasy is so powerful to us. When combined with machine learning, our favorite websites are constantly surprising us with more of what we like. It's like a slot machine in our brain.

The effect is so strong it even tricks our physiology. Known as the Coolidge effect, it's been observed in nature that males who display a declining interest in mating with the same female over time will show heightened sexual interest when new females are introduced.

In my own pursuit of porn, even when I was tired and needed to sleep, I would stay on computers for hours driven by the endless searching.

---

5. Blaise Pascal, *Pensees* (Mineola, New York: Dover Publications, 2003), 40.

LOVE AND BELONGING

One of the biggest reasons that people get stuck in porn is they feel isolated. We might have a family or a wife who loves us, but we're struggling to receive that love and stay connected. And again, we're going to porn to deal with our needs to feel like we belong. But porn actually heightens our sense of isolation and disconnection. This is why we're left feeling crappy after acting out. Because we've withdrawn to act out, we feel shame and guilt, which makes it harder for us to connect. Intimacy and deep friendship or even sexual intimacy with our spouse or partner becomes harder when we're continuing to go to this false source of love.

Heavy pornography use could be a sign of an intimacy disorder. We're looking for love and belonging in our porn and, of course, it's never going to give us that. We sense a deficit in ourselves, and we go to porn as a way to meet that need instead of getting it from the people in our life.

SELF-ESTEEM

How does esteem affect us in porn?

We want to feel good enough, we want to feel affirmed, we want to feel valued. We want to feel important.

Sometimes guys resist this need thinking it's like narcissism. But it's more like the need of a small child who rightly craves the healthy attention of his parents. He looks to his primary care givers for his sense of worth and confidence. We need this too.

This particular need is really expressed in our hunger for porn. It goes beyond just the sense of love and belonging. We want this praise and esteem at a high level.

We use porn not only as a way to feel affirmed, but as a way to get confidence. We're in control when we're looking at the porn. We feel empowered.

Of course, when it's over, we realize that it's a false empowerment. It's a false confidence. It doesn't last; it's temporal.

SELF-ACTUALIZATION

Physiological, safety, love and belonging, esteem—those are all things we need, and we're trying to meet those needs with porn. The last need that Maslow talks about is self-actualization. This need doesn't come out of deprivation, but comes out of a desire to grow, to meet one's full potential.

It has to do with collaborating with others. We are no longer "giving to get" because our primary needs are met. We instead are free to be our true selves serving our community and being fully present with those in our life. We can see the good in others and call it out.

No, porn never lets us get to this point because it doesn't meet our needs. We are still running at a deficit.

But the need is there none the less. If you picked up this book, you know you are called to something more. That there is potential that's not being realized in your life, and you want more.

SO WHAT IS SELF-CARE?

It's your system for identifying your needs and meeting them. A few chapters back, I mentioned threats. In our after-action reviews, we are looking ahead for situations where we need tools. It's easy to only think of these as tempting situations. Things involving porn, lust, fantasy, etc. These are most acute in early recovery.

But your long-term success will be determined by how you recognize and meet deep needs consistently. That is the essence of self-care.

Rather than ramble on about this and that, I have created some questions to help prompt you for each set of needs.

PHYSIOLOGICAL

- Are you getting enough sleep?
- What do you need to do to keep up your physical health?
- How's your diet?
- Are you brushing, flossing, showering?

SAFETY

- Are you taking unnecessary risks?
- Is your home environment safe?
- Are there any situations or places you feel the need to avoid?
- Are there any nonessential apps or devices you need to get rid of?
- Are there certain times a day you would benefit from limiting screen time?
- Do you need a filter or accountability?
- Could your work station be less private?
- Do you need to create some boundaries with technology, with work, with people?

VARIETY / UNCERTAINTY

- What are you looking forward to?
- If I looked at your calendar, would you have something fun scheduled?
- How do you find adventure?

- What are you learning?
- What's a passion you have that doesn't involve a screen?
- Where are you being creative?
- What sports or competition do you have in your life?

LOVE AND BELONGING

- Where do you find belonging and community?
- Where can you be yourself?
- If you're in a relationship, how can you create more safety and intimacy with your partner?
- If you have kids, what can you do to create more connection and be present for them?

ESTEEM

- Who in your life encourages you?
- Where can you be honest without receiving judgment?
- Who are you helping? Who's helping you?
- Who are you serving?
- Who can speak the truth to you?

SELF-ACTUALIZATION

- Where are you growing?
- Where do you find your greatest meaning in life?
- What does giving up porn make possible for you?
- Who inspires you?
- Who are you collaborating with?
- What's next for you?

CHAPTER 9

BECOMING THE TYPE OF MAN WHO DOES NOT LOOK AT PORN

ONE OF THE MOST AMAZING PARTS OF MY work is getting to see guys do recovery in real time. One of the most memorable correspondences I have had with a podcast listener is below.

A man named Jon messaged me:

Hey Matt, I love the Porn Free Radio show, and it has been an instrumental part of helping with my recovery. I took your advice and created a recovery plan, and as of today I'm on day 81 P/M free! Keep up the important work you are doing, it makes a difference!

When guys share with me a streak, I love to find out more. I replied:

Wow, that is great to hear. What's been working for you? Any a-ha moments that helped you move forward?

His response:

The "ah-ha" moment for me was perhaps more of a progressive epiphany. When I first started my journey, I was studying lots of porn-based literature, studies, No fap blogging, podcast listening, etc.

And while I still do those things, they are measurably less, as I have concerted my efforts into a different focus. That focus being daily investment in building my character.

I know you are familiar with The Miracle Morning by Hal Elrod, and that has become my daily routine.

I spend approximately 100 minutes every morning to start each day: reading, writing, meditating, affirmations, visualization, exercise, and thanksgiving.

The turning point for me with recovery came with the realization that "what you behold is what you become." And that if my focus is constantly on porn, even if its recovery steps and literature, that I would always be in "recovery," as opposed to being "recovered."

I am inhabiting a place of "becoming the type of man that does not look at porn." Instead of "practicing behaviors that keep me from looking at porn."

I find that becoming the man naturally aligns my character, and I am therefore inhabiting that behavior.

I think those are diametrically different approaches to recovery. I am focusing on who I am becoming. And as a result, I am living as that man. It is no longer a daily struggle for me of battling temptation, avoidance behavior, hobby enthusiasm, or the like.

This was and is my breakthrough.

This inspires me today. Jon nails something that is important to us moving forward.

We can't recover with just porn-avoiding strategies. Recovery is active. We need something to replace not only that time with, but the identity we relate to. Like the hundred minutes every morning where Jon's reading, and writing, and having thanksgiving, and exercise.

I ask guys all the time what their plan is. I am hoping to hear about some cool activities, but inevitably someone starts talking about, "Well, I have this filtered, and I have this cut off, and I don't do this, and I don't do that." It's a laundry list of all these things he doesn't do. A set of rigid rules. There's no energy in that.

I do a coaching exercise where I ask guys, "What are you moving toward?"

And guys inevitably will say, "Well, I don't want to feel shame anymore," or "I don't want to feel controlled by my addiction anymore."

But all the things that they think they're moving toward are negative: *not* feeling something, something *not* happening.

And I'll ask, "Can you think of a positive way to say that? What does it mean to live without shame? What's the opposite of that? Is it contentment? Is it being okay in your own skin? Is it having integrity?"

When I put a destination in my phone GPS. I first want to know what direction to go. Then I need prompts along the way to keep me on course. Finally, I need to know when I arrive at my destination.

Can you imagine if our GPS just focused on our starting point?

You are 93 miles away from Chicago.
You have been driving for 82 minutes.
You have been driving on Interstate 94.

Many of us backed into recovery. We get caught by our wives or had a rock-bottom moment that scared us. We don't feel confident, we don't feel energized, and we actually feel scared.

And we react from that place. We clamp down. We make resolutions about what we're *not* going to do, what we're going to get rid of. We're going to get rid of our iPhone, or we're going to put a filter on, or we will never go to that website again.

We're scrambling to get out of danger. It's basic survival. Many of us start recovery that way, and it makes sense. But it's not sustainable. Once the feeling of immediate danger passes, we slip back.

We're not just recovering from something; we're recovering *to* something. I love where Jon puts his focus. He's focusing his efforts on investing in his character, investing in the man who he wants to be.

That doesn't mean we don't have boundaries; it doesn't mean that we don't use tools to deal with pornography. But simply not doing something can't be the *only* focus.

My friend Scott put it this way. He's a mountain biker, and he noticed this pattern when he went down a trail fast. If he focused on the trail and where he was going, he would stay on the path, but if he ever put too much focus on a rock he wanted to avoid, he would instinctively start driving toward it. Whatever he put his focus on is what he ended up moving toward.

When we put our focus on who we want to be, on who we're becoming, we're likely to hit it. If we put our focus only on the porn—even if we're focusing on it to avoid it—we're likely to hit it. Jon reminds us, "What you behold is what you become."

If all we focus on is what we don't do, that becomes our focus. It's not full living, it's not the whole picture.

I no longer refer to myself as a porn addict. I also don't refer to the guys I work with as porn addicts. When you say someone's a porn addict, it makes it seem like a definitive statement, like this is who they are forever.

Instead, I prefer focusing on who you're becoming, and making that your primary identity, making that transformation the thing you're moving toward.

I am sure this is a little ironic coming from the Porn Free guy. I spend a lot of time talking about porn. But I don't identify with the idea of being a porn addict anymore. I am a recovered man who hasn't looked at porn since January 2011.

Do I still have the weakness? Are there things that I can be tempted by? Are there places where I still need tools? Absolutely. Those things are true, and yet I'm a different person than I was when I was looking at porn every day.

A. W. Tozer refers to this process of becoming. He writes,

> "We are all in the process of becoming. We have already moved from what we were to what we are, and we are now moving toward

what we shall be. The perturbing thought is not that we are becoming, but what we are becoming; not that we are moving; but toward what we are moving. We are becoming what we love."[1]

I love this idea. Whether we like it or not, we're moving, we're becoming. We're moving from what we were to what we are, and we're moving toward what we're going to be.

There is no use wondering about whether we're moving. We are. It's often said that not to act is to act. You know? If we get stuck, if we procrastinate, we're still making a choice.

"We are becoming what we love," Tozer writes.

So we have to grapple with this question: What do we love? If we no longer are going to porn, where is our focus? What do we value? What do we love? Integrity? People? Healthy relationships?

I love this idea of inhabiting the place, of becoming the type of man who does not look at porn.

Get a picture of a healthy guy who doesn't look at porn. What does he value in life? What does he pursue so that porn doesn't take up that healthy place in his life? What does he value?

Now, I'm not perfect, but I've become a man who doesn't look at porn. So, what do I do with my time?

---

1. A. W. Tozer, *God Tells the Man Who Cares* (Chicago: Moody Publishers, 1993).

I have more space in my life. I do more self-care, like a morning writing routine. I've worked on getting healthier with food and fitness. I've started a business. I read lots of books. I have been involved in recovery groups. I've started groups to help others. I've started a podcast and write to help others. I still go to therapy. I have one-on-one accountability relationships. I do check-ins with my wife. I am more creative than ever and do lots of things that would've scared me in the past.

"I am focusing on who I am becoming," Jon concludes. "And as a result, I am living as that man."

One critical habit Jon has added is daily contact with a group of guys through text. He connects and encourages other guys to step up. Those habits sustain long-term recovery.

So, who are you without porn?

I have an Evernote file called *Stuff Matt Likes*.

I know it sounds strange, but when we are dependent on porn, it dulls us to the things that bring us joy and curiosity in our lives.

The file has grown as I add new interests and remember things I liked as a kid. Skateboarding, old-school rap music, dancing on jumbotrons, Hallmark Christmas movies, and the Ramones are all on the list.

When I was a kid, we were in a church with a great preacher, Jimmy Young. Even as a third-grader, I was inspired by the dramatic way he taught. He would get so into it, he would bang on the pulpit.

A few years back I looked him up and found out his church podcasts all his sermons. I started listening and he was as good as I remember.

In one of the sermons, he mentioned a weekend Bible class he teaches every summer in Memphis, Tennessee. I added that to my list.

After some careful planning and a lot of emails to Dr. Young's assistant, I traveled from Chicago to Memphis in 2019. It was amazing.

That's a small example of following and cultivating your passions.

I have dozens of other examples. Starting a ministry to help others. Losing weight. Getting a promotion at work. Starting a podcast. Starting a business. Writing this book!

All were made possible by the space that was freed up in my life by letting go of porn.

Coach Craig Perra says, "Success comes from 50 percent recovery work and 50 percent kicking ass in life."[2]

Even now, it's easy for me to focus on the struggle. The boundaries I have to keep. The habits I have to maintain to stay porn free.

---

2. Craig Perra, The Mindful Habit, https://www.themindfulhabit
.com/about-craig-perra/.

But then I think what am I doing to kick ass in life? What excites me? What sparks joy?

I was writing in a French coffee shop a few months back. They had a special on macarons.

Macarons are colorful little pastries that taste like a cloud of sugar. The line was out the door with customers waiting to buy them. Even though the line was long, everyone was smiling, anticipating eating the macarons.

Once they got them, they were taking pictures for their Instagram and sharing tastes with one another. It was pure joy. I need this too!

What am I waiting in line for? What am I anticipating? What makes me smile?

We have to enlarge our vision. "What might freedom be for?" asks author Jay Stringer. "Why do you want to be free?"[3]

I recently was a guest on a podcast. The interviewer was a former college film professor. He asked if I was sad that there were some movies that I couldn't watch because they were triggering or overly sexual.

I used to think like this, that I was cutting off all the fun in life. All the good movies. All the TV shows people talked about at work. But I realized there is

3. Jay Stringer, *Unwanted: How Sexual Brokenness Reveals Our Way to Healing* (Colorado Springs: The Navigators, 2018).

still a whole world of things that I can pursue. My life is rich, and I find many things that I can enjoy.

"If your hope is not moving your story into a greater passion and comfort," Jay Stringer writes. "Your desire for freedom is too small."[4]

Is your desire too small? Do you have a small vision for recovery?

I hear guys all the time resigning themselves to a lifetime of struggle and disappointment. It doesn't have to be that way.

We were made for more joy. More fulfilment. More desire. More happiness.

I agree with C. S. Lewis when he says, "It would seem that Our Lord finds our desires not too strong, but too weak."[5]

The pursuit of porn is not a strong desire, it's weak. It's a distraction, a mirage. Real recovery doesn't stifle desire, it liberates it.

Take hope and take action.

4. Jay Stringer, *Unwanted: How Sexual Brokenness Reveals Our Way to Healing* (Colorado Springs: The Navigators, 2018).
5. C. S. Lewis, *The Weight of Glory* (United Kingdom: HarperCollins, 2001), 26.

APPENDIX
YOUR WHY

YOU STARTED THIS PROCESS, BUT DO YOU know why?

I became a runner a few years ago. After years of sedentary living, I had embraced a new habit. I was running daily. I ran a few 5Ks. My goal was to run a 5K in under thirty minutes. It was something I had always wanted to do, but some self-limiting beliefs kept me from it. When I finally started doing it, I loved it.

But, like most new runners, I got injured. After seeing a physical therapist and a knee expert, I was instructed to stop running until my leg could heal. I had to train using my bike. I hated it because I wanted to run. To make matters worse, in my area, there are a lot of bikers who wear spandex and special outfits, and I would judge them. I didn't want to be like them. I'm a runner. I would feel sorry for myself as I rode down the bike path by the lake. I was jealous when I would see runners because I was stuck on my bike.

My trainer noticed this pattern where I was exercising but resentful. She had me memorize a phrase: *I am riding my bike so I can run again.* She said, "I want you to say this every time you're tempted to feel sorry for yourself, anytime you see a runner on the bike path that you're jealous of, or anytime you see a biker in spandex that you just can't stand. I want you to say, 'I'm riding my bike so I can run again.'"

I needed a clear reminder of why I was doing this. It had to be something I could easily recall in the moment when I was upset, when I was triggered, or when I felt resentful. Something to remind me what the bigger purpose of riding my bike was.

What Friedrich Nietzsche says is true: "He who has a why to live for can bear almost any how."[1]

I don't know about you, but I take some hope in that quote. If we can get laser focused and zero in on what your "why" is, then I'm confident that you can endure any of the changes that need to take place in your life to make it happen.

So why are you doing this? Many of the guys I coach answer this question like this: my wife, my

---

1. Friedrich Nietzsche, as quoted by Viktor Emil Frankl, *Man's Search for Meaning* (United Kingdom: Beacon Press, 1992), 109.

marriage. You may have been caught by your wife downloading pornography. Maybe it's come up in your marriage. It's a point of conflict. Other guys talk about their job or their ministry. Maybe you've been caught viewing pornography at your job. Or maybe you're scared of being caught. Or maybe you're in conflict with your ministry or your faith.

Other guys mention kids, family, etc. That's another important motivation. Those are all good reasons, but they're all external. For your why, we have to go deeper.

What's in it for *you* to go porn free? Not your wife, not somebody else—what's in it for you? What's your selfish reason for quitting porn? What do you get out it?

I have an exercise to help us determine what your "why" is. I learned this method from two business coaches, Jason Van Orden and Jeremy Frandsen. They referred to it as a single, motivating purpose. We need to get clear what our single, motivating purpose is for doing anything in life. This is especially true with going porn free.

Take out a piece of paper and draw a line down the middle. On one side write **Costs**, and on the other side, write **Benefits**.

For the costs, write down everything porn costs you. What are the direct and indirect costs of you engaging with porn? Think about what stings the most. The more specific you can get the better.

Really dial in what you are sick of when it comes to your porn use?

Take a few minutes to make your list.

Then, under benefits, I want you to imagine that we had a magic wand and we can eliminate porn from your life. What would the immediate benefits be? What would some of the long-term benefits be?

As you think about the benefits don't just write down the opposite of the costs. If you write down loss of confidence as a cost, don't just write confidence as a benefit. Instead ask the question, "If I had the confidence porn has taken from me, what would I do with it? Who would I be? What would the benefit be?"

You might be surprised what comes out of those questions.

Example Costs:

- loss of trust
- destroys my confidence
- loss of time
- shame
- money
- feeling out of control
- feeling like a hypocrite
- makes me numb

Example Benefits:

- able to receive and give love
- joy (contentment)
- feeling of freedom
- the same on the inside as on the outside
- more present with my family
- capacity to achieve big goals

After you've finished, I want you to look at them all again. Review the costs. Zero in on the number one thing you are most sick and tired of.

Of all the benefits you wrote down, identify which one makes you think, "Hell yes! If I could get that I would be thrilled. That's what I want."

Circle one idea in each column. Maybe the shame is the thing you're sick of. You're tired of always feeling like you're never good enough or that you're broken.

For the benefit, you might choose joy. It's that feeling of contentment or being okay in your own skin. That's what you want to move toward.

Keep these ideas in mind as we craft your why statement.

This statement will crystallize exactly why you're doing this and serves as a good reminder, like the reminder I had when I was training.

Your why include two things: *a cost of pornography* and a specific *benefit to quitting.*

Let's put them together in this sentence:

I'm committed to being porn free because I'm tired of [specific cost], and I want more [specific benefit] in my life.

Example:

I'm committed to being porn free because I'm tired of living with shame and I want more joy in my life.

This type of sentence can be powerful. You're not quitting because of something external (i.e., your wife, your job, your church). Instead, you are engaging your internal motivation. When we create a WHY with a cost we are tired of and a powerful benefit we want to move toward, we set up two poles in our life: a relapse pole where we remind ourselves about the cost of acting out, and a recovery pole where we begin to focus on the benefit of being porn free.

SHAME  **JOY**

We are always in a state of movement. I love the quote, "We are either working on recovery, or working on relapse." At any given time, we are headed in one direction or the other. This is especially true when we're actively making choices.

- If you're hiding some unsound activity . . . you're heading back to living in Shame
- Establishing a new morning routine . . . moving toward Joy
- Skipping your men's group because you feel good . . . Shame
- Planning a date night for your wife . . . Joy
- Creating a recovery plan and activating it . . . Joy
- Circumventing your safety measures . . . Shame

To inspire you, here are some real examples from other guys . . .

- I'm tired of being numb and I want to actively pursue a great life.
- I'm tired of self-hatred and mediocre living and I want confidence and the capacity to achieve big goals.
- I'm tired of wrecking my self-confidence and I want to be an expert in my field.
- I'm tired of living with a burden of guilt and I want real joy.
- I'm tired of being stuck and distracted and I want to execute on my dreams.

And my all-time favorite which is metaphorical but awesome . . .

- I'm committed to being porn free because I'm tired of living off of chicken nuggets and french fries, and I want more ski slopes, Hulk rides, and BBQ in my life."

Create a WHY that fits you!

ACTION

Over the next 24 hours, I want you to repeat your WHY at least 10 times. Get it down in your memory. What are you tired of? What do you want? Memorize it. Say it out loud at least 10 times. Write it out, too, so you get really confident saying it. If you wrote down a lot of words, reduce it and make it simple. Get it as clear and concise as possible.

Be prepared to share this WHY with someone else. Get comfortable saying it to others, but I also want you to internalize why you're going through this process. Say it out loud to yourself often.

I want you to repeat it, especially when you experience craving. If you're discouraged or you start feeling despair like you can't do this or you're feeling down, remind yourself of your single motivating purpose.

Finally, as you become aware of threats (situations that need tools) remind yourself of your WHY. It could be something as simple as realizing you *need to stop watching a TV show with triggers or needing to close a browser window because the site you're on is heading toward relapse. You need to ask yourself why am I doing this? Ask yourself, which way am I headed?*

Repeat your WHY.

SMALL GROUP DISCUSSION QUESTIONS

INTRODUCTION

1. The opening story is about a "wake-up call" that David experienced around his porn usage (and the consequences he saw for others). Have you experienced a wake-up call around your porn usage? If so, in what way?

2. The author says his podcast (and this book) is for "motivated guys who want to quit looking at porn." Where would you place your level of motivation on the scale below and why?

1	5	9
Wondering if this is a problem	Growing realization that things need to change	Fully aware and motivated

3. The introduction describes how David had a number of unsuccessful attempts to walk away from porn that undermined his confidence. What efforts have you made to walk away from porn in your life? How successful have these efforts been, and how does this affect your confidence regarding your ability to change?

CHAPTER 1: BEING ALONE

1. When was the first time you remember seeing porn? What were the feelings associated with that experience?

2. If you received a message about porn or masturbation from your parents, what was that message?

3. The author speaks about a "disconnect" between his faith/values and his growing porn behaviors. Did this disconnect happen for you, and if so, how would you describe it?

4. The author speaks about the feeling of isolation and shame that surrounded his porn struggle and then the experience of being "seen" by someone. How "seen" have you felt in your struggle? What steps have you taken to become

"known"? Where would you place yourself on this continuum and why?

1	5	9
Still mostly locked away	Taking some early steps	Been "seen" for a while

5. The author describes the experience of being "alone" as a major trigger in his early childhood. Can you think of a feeling that leaves you vulnerable to wanting to run to porn?

CHAPTER 2: THE PORN SOLUTION

1. Which of the following "problem" messages have you heard about porn?

_____ It is a sin against God.

_____ It is something we should hate.

_____ It is bad for your brain.

_____ It is a sign of poor self-discipline or self-control.

_____ It is a drug that turns us into addicts.

_____ It is a spiritual battle for purity we must win.

_____ It is a weakness of our flesh that must be overcome.

2. The above statements may contain elements of truth but also can lead us to a brutal hangover every time we act out. If any of the following words resonate with you, add some short statements underneath with things you have felt or told yourself around your struggle with porn.

Shame:

_____

_____

Helplessness:

_____

_____

Hopelessness:

_____

_____

3. The author makes a provocative statement: "Porn is not the problem for us; it is the solution." What is your first reaction when you hear that statement?

4. What are some problems you try to solve with porn?

5. If recovery is the process of getting healthy (and not just avoiding at porn), what are some of the areas in your life that you need to address?

CHAPTER 3: BUT WAIT, ISN'T PORN AN ADDICTION?

1. What feelings do you associate with the idea of porn being an addiction and you being an addict? (There may be a variety of opinions here!)

2. Does your perspective on addiction change if you see it as an "extreme version of a habit"? If so, how?

3. What are some of the costs that you associate with your porn habit?

4. The author outlines four ways that porn robs us of time. For each of the four, describe how this has felt to you.

Porn's Effects	My Experience
It dishonors my value	
It spontaneously overrides my life	
It ruins my next day	
It robs me of my presence	

Now describe what your life would look and feel like without the effects above.

_____

_____

_____

_____

_____

5. The author ends the chapter using the story of the *Cloven Viscount* to illustrate that wholeness is the goal of your recovery. What does integrity and wholeness mean to you? What do you make of the author's suggestion that we need to move beyond simply seeing ourself as having a "good side" and a "bad side" and move toward a more "integrated approach"?

CHAPTER 4: EITHER WE GET CAUGHT OR WE GET COURAGE

1. Was your desire to get porn out of your life prompted by getting caught or did it come from a desire to change on your own? Do you think it makes a difference? If so, why?

2. Early in our recovery, we break through shame and isolation by stepping into honesty and exposure. Describe how this has felt to you.

3. The author describes three reasons why we avoid taking the steps above: looking bad, aversion of loss, and fear of pain. What are the reasons that have kept you in isolation and hiddenness?

4. The author describes three gifts of being known: no more hiding, the ability to focus on the real problem, and the opportunity to experience love and acceptance. In what ways have you experienced these gifts?

5. "Every man needs help and every man has some help to give" (Nate Larkin). What are the benefits of being in a group of like-minded men—who share your struggles but are also motived to lead more integrated and healthy lives?

CHAPTER 5: THE DARK NIGHT

1. In reading the author's description of his dark night, can you relate to any aspects of this story? If you have experienced this "darkness," how would you describe it?

2. What or who have you blamed for your difficulties in putting porn aside in your life?

3. The author describes the "pushback" or "power-shift" he experienced when he started out on his desired journey to live a new way. How does this "resistance" show up in your recovery journey?

CHAPTER 6: THE PORN FREE PLAN THAT NEVER FAILS

1. What is your first thought when you see the title of this chapter: hope, skepticism, or something else?

2. Ask yourself this question: *On a scale of one to nine, where would I place myself on the awareness that porn is no longer working for me?*

1 _____ **9**

It's not that big of a deal   It's killing me!

3. If denial is a mechanism we use to avoid the uncomfortable truth of our situation, what are some of the excuses you have made for keeping porn in your life?

4. The author says there is a big difference between awareness and deciding to change. What keeps you from being ready to take the actual steps to become porn free? (For example, you could be one that confuses "research" with taking action.)

5. What makes it hard for you to connect with others about your porn habits? (You can check more than one.)

    ____ The belief that "I take care of me"
    ____ I don't want to look bad
    ____ Shame/embarrassment
    ____ My situation is unique (so others wouldn't understand)
    ____ Vulnerability is hard for me
    ____ Previously bad experiences in something like this
    ____ I want God to take care of it (because He should know me)
    ____ Create your own: _____

    _____

6. What is "Your Why" for wanting to quit porn? (For help with this question, complete the exercise in the book's appendix located immediately after chapter 9.)

7. What are the emotional triggers and mistaken beliefs that come before you wanting to look at porn?

8. What are some simple, practical ways that you could remove weak links in your technology that leave you vulnerable to craving?

9. What do you think of the idea of porn as an extreme habit rather than an "addiction"? Do you think the idea of creating a different "system" of habits is one that could work in your favor? Explain.

10. What are three new active commitments you could use to begin unleashing the power of positive habits?

    1. _____

    2. _____

    3. _____

11. What is one way that you could celebrate steady movement toward your goal? (Set a goal of 1-week or 1-month porn free to start.)

    (reward) _____

    _____

12. What is one way that you could remind yourself (not punish yourself) with a consequence if you choose porn over completing your goal?

(consequence) _____

_____

13. Who could you share your plan with as a way of activating it in your life?

14. Why is reviewing and improving our recovery plan necessary? How does the F.A.S.T. check-in listed in the chapter remind us of this basic truth?

CHAPTER 7: THE ENEMY OF RECOVERY IS SELF-REJECTION

1. From the author's story, we see that children are great recorders but lousy interpreters. Can you think of an early event in your life where your interpretation has left you with ongoing false beliefs about yourself or others?

2. Based on the previous question, what set of unmet needs could still be in play in your life?

3. What coping mechanisms and strategies have you used to to meet your unmet needs?

4. Can you think of any ways that you practice "self-rejection"?

5. What difference would it make for you if, at the core of your being, you believed that you are "beloved"?

CHAPTER 8: SELF-CARE

1. When you think of self-care, what comes to mind?

2. How do you beat yourself up after a relapse?

3. In what way has porn been "unhealthy self-care" for you? (Think about the needs it promises to meet.)

4. The author talks about his favorite chair. Do you have a location that you identify with as your place of self-care?

5. Where in your life do you feel "out of control" or unsafe?

6. Do you identify with the author when he says that there is a part of us that longs for "escape, excitement, or adventure"? What are the things in life that activate this desire for you?

7. Take some time and work through the questions that the author includes for each of the below areas. Jot down any key insights that could help you create both equilibrium and health in your life.

   - Physiological
   - Safety
   - Variety/Uncertainty
   - Love and Belonging
   - Esteem
   - Self-Actualization

CHAPTER 9: BECOMING THE TYPE OF MAN WHO DOES NOT LOOK AT PORN

1. What do you see as the difference between "practicing behaviors that keep me from looking at porn" and "becoming the type of man who does not look at porn"?

2. How would you answer the question, "What are you moving toward?"

3. In regard to your response for the previous question, do you feel that your daily activities support the ongoing movement in this direction?

4. Do you think that your reasons for wanting to be free from porn have evolved over time? If so, in what way? From this chapter, what would you say you would like your long-term motivation to be based on?

5. What are some new (or old) passions that you would like to cultivate to replace the role porn used to occupy in your life?

6. Describe the hope you have taken from reading this book.

7. What is an action you will take as a result?

8. Finally, who could help you take this action?

ACKNOWLEDGMENTS

"It is *for* freedom that Christ has set us free."

—Galatians 5:1 (NIV)

WE WERE MADE TO LIVE IN FREEDOM, NOT bondage.

And God used a lot unique people to help me get free from porn, which is what made this book possible.

To my gracious wife, Janice . . . Thank you. Your love and support, when I didn't deserve it, is what broke open my heart for greater freedom.

There are others, too, who encouraged me along the way . . .

Thanks to Judy-Rae, Charles, Mario, Andy, Amy, John, Cheryll, Steve, Lis, Burt, Kati, Little Amy, and Mark.

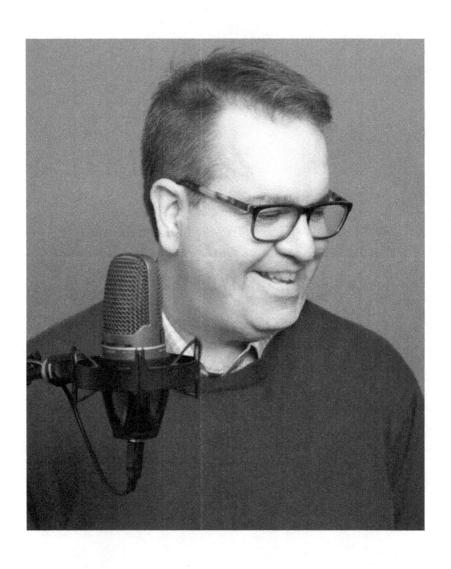

ABOUT THE AUTHOR

MATT DOBSCHUETZ IS THE HOST OF Porn Free Radio, the top-rated podcast for motivated guys who want to quit looking at porn. His hope-filled approach to a subject many have trouble talking about has inspired a global audience of men to take action and transform their lives. From his home in suburban Chicago, Matt podcasts and runs a professional coaching practice. He is happily married to his wife, Janice, with whom he has been friends since college. Together, they have two teenage sons. Matt is a diehard Chicago Bears fan, a coffee enthusiast, and a lover of old-school hip hop.

I WOULD APPRECIATE YOUR FEEDBACK ON WHAT CHAPTERS HELPED YOU MOST AND WHAT YOU WOULD LIKE TO SEE IN FUTURE BOOKS.

IF YOU ENJOYED THIS BOOK AND FOUND IT HELPFUL, PLEASE LEAVE A **REVIEW** ON AMAZON.

VISIT ME AT

WWW.PORNFREEBOOK.COM

WHERE YOU CAN SIGN UP FOR EMAIL UPDATES.

THANK YOU!

Printed in the USA
CPSIA information can be obtained
at www.ICGtesting.com
LVHW041955101023
760757LV00003B/402